BREAK THE MOLD

BREAK THE MOLD

5 Tools To Conquer Mold and Take Back Your Health

Dr. Jill Crista

Wellness Ink Publishing

Break The Mold
5 Tools to Conquer Mold and Take Back Your Health

Wellness Ink Publishing | www.WellnessInk.com
ISBN: 978-1-988645-18-6 (paperback) | ISBN: 978-1-988645-19-3 (e-book)
Cover and interior design | Kristin Hodgkinson
support@drcrista.com | www.drcrista.com

Quantity discounts and customized versions are available for bulk purchases. For permission requests or quantity discounts, please email support@drcrista.com.

Dedication

To the remediation crews that healed my home.
I'll be ever indebted for the rescue, your kindness, and patience.
The work you do is life-saving.

CONTENTS

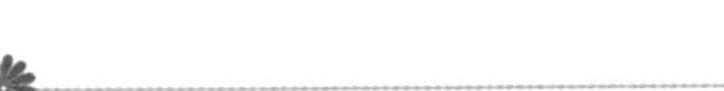
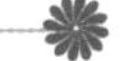

Crista Mold Questionnaire

Date Taken

CHECK **ALL SYMPTOMS** EXPERIENCED IN THE **PAST 3-6 MONTHS**

For a printable copy of this questionnaire, send an email request to support@drcrista.com.

CATEGORY 1

- ☐ Brain fog
- ☐ Feel tired all the time
- ☐ Frequent runny nose
- ☐ Blow your nose often
- ☐ Sneezing
- ☐ Sinusitis
- ☐ Post-nasal drip
- ☐ Nose bleeds
- ☐ Swollen glands
- ☐ Shortness of breath
- ☐ Frequent yawning or sighing
- ☐ Heart palpitations
- ☐ Headaches
- ☐ Hay fever
- ☐ Eye irritation
- ☐ Blurry vision
- ☐ Frequent change in vision
- ☐ Allergies
- ☐ Dark circles under eyes
- ☐ Sensitivity to sunlight
- ☐ Nervousness/can't settle
- ☐ Low mood or depressed
- ☐ Feeling overwhelmed
- ☐ Episodic/chronic dry cough
- ☐ Irritated lungs
- ☐ Blood-streaked mucous
- ☐ Nasal polyps
- ☐ Coated tongue
- ☐ Sores in the mouth
- ☐ Bumps on back of throat
- ☐ Thrush
- ☐ Sore or itchy ear canals
- ☐ Ringing in the ears
- ☐ Bothered by loud noises
- ☐ Skin rash
- ☐ Burning or itchy skin
- ☐ Easy bruising
- ☐ Spider veins
- ☐ Bothered by tags and seams on clothing
- ☐ Anemia
- ☐ Protruding veins on limbs
- ☐ Lower extremity edema
- ☐ Clear your throat often
- ☐ Sore throat
- ☐ Frequent colds
- ☐ Delayed recovery from colds
- ☐ Exhausted from exercise
- ☐ Frequent static shocks
- ☐ Increased thirst
- ☐ Trouble sleeping
- ☐ Feeling of internal vibration
- ☐ Dizziness
- ☐ Vertigo
- ☐ Drunken feeling
- ☐ Frequent urination
- ☐ Yeast infection
- ☐ Change in appetite
- ☐ Intestinal gas
- ☐ Nausea
- ☐ Feeling bloated
- ☐ Constipation
- ☐ Crave sweets
- ☐ Crave alcohol

TOTAL **CATEGORY 1** BOXES MARKED: ________

0-4 boxes marked = Score 0
5-9 boxes marked = Score 1
10-15 boxes marked = Score 2
16+ boxes marked = Score 3

CATEGORY **1** SCORE ______

Continue to Category 2

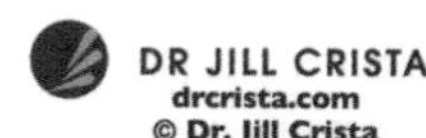

Crista Mold Questionnaire continued

CHECK **ALL SYMPTOMS** EXPERIENCED IN THE **PAST 3-6 MONTHS**

CATEGORY **2**

- ☐ Wheezing
- ☐ Asthma
- ☐ Burning lungs
- ☐ Recurrent respiratory infections
- ☐ Migraine
- ☐ Allergies aren't well controlled by medication
- ☐ Voice sounds nasally
- ☐ Plugged or clogged ears
- ☐ Chronic sinusitis
- ☐ Vomiting
- ☐ Alternating constipation/ diarrhea
- ☐ Diarrhea
- ☐ Irritable bowel
- ☐ Food sensitivities
- ☐ Chemical sensitivities
- ☐ Abnormal reaction to antibiotics
- ☐ Epstein-Barr virus
- ☐ Recurrent yeast infections
- ☐ Bacterial vaginosis
- ☐ Recurrent athlete's foot, jock itch, or toenail fungus
- ☐ Peeling/sloughing skin
- ☐ Episodes of fast heart rate
- ☐ Chest pain
- ☐ Raynaud's syndrome
- ☐ Non-obstructive sleep apnea
- ☐ Difficulty thinking clearly
- ☐ Disorientation
- ☐ Balance Issues
- ☐ Slow reflexes
- ☐ Incoordination
- ☐ Numbness or tingling
- ☐ Nerve pains
- ☐ Unexplained menstrual changes
- ☐ Overactive bladder
- ☐ Bladder infection
- ☐ React to musty spaces

TOTAL **CATEGORY 2** BOXES MARKED: ______

0-2 boxes marked = Score 0
3-5 boxes marked = Score 1
6-9 boxes marked = Score 2
10+ boxes marked = Score 3

CATEGORY **2** SCORE ______

Continue to Category 3

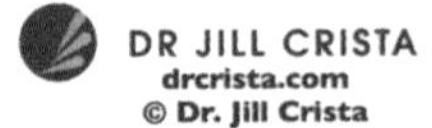

Crista Mold Questionnaire continued

CHECK **ALL SYMPTOMS** EXPERIENCED IN THE **PAST 3-6 MONTHS**

CATEGORY **3**

- ☐ Daily use of sinus spray, sinus prescription, or Neti pot
- ☐ Sinus surgery at any time in your life
- ☐ Chronic inflammatory response syndrome (CIRS)
- ☐ MARCoNS
- ☐ Peanut allergy
- ☐ Chronic fatigue syndrome
- ☐ Difficulty walking
- ☐ Dysautonomia
- ☐ Postural Tachycardia Syndrome (PoTS)
- ☐ Hearing loss
- ☐ Confusion
- ☐ Dementia
- ☐ Memory loss
- ☐ Tremors
- ☐ Sarcoidosis
- ☐ Asthma that's difficult to control with medication
- ☐ Idiopathic pneumonitis
- ☐ Lung scarring or nodules
- ☐ Respiratory distress
- ☐ Aspergillosis
- ☐ Arrhythmia
- ☐ Coagulation abnormalities
- ☐ Atriovenous abnormalities
- ☐ Churg Strauss Syndrome
- ☐ Histamine intolerance
- ☐ Erythema nodosum
- ☐ Eosinophilic esophagitis
- ☐ Ulcer
- ☐ Non-celiac intestinal disease
- ☐ Blood in stool
- ☐ Cyclical vomiting syndrome
- ☐ Liver pain or swelling
- ☐ Fatty liver
- ☐ Non-alcoholic steatohepatitis (NASH)
- ☐ Interstitial cystitis
- ☐ Kidney pain or swelling
- ☐ Kidney disease
- ☐ Nephritis
- ☐ Chronic pelvic pain
- ☐ Infertility
- ☐ Hepatocellular carcinoma
- ☐ Previous or current cancer diagnosis
- ☐ Mast cell activation syndrome (MCAS)
- ☐ Exposure to water-damaged building any time in your life
- ☐ Exposure to mold
- ☐ Positive Shoemaker tests

TOTAL **CATEGORY 3** BOXES MARKED: ______

Score 1 for each box marked
Boxes marked and score will be the same for this category

CATEGORY **3** SCORE ______

Continue to Results

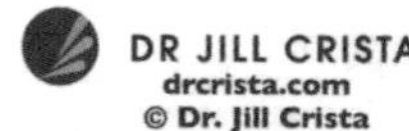

TOTAL MOLD RISK **RESULTS**

Gather your Category scores
from the 3 previous pages

CATEGORY 1 SCORE: ______ +
CATEGORY 2 SCORE: ______ +
CATEGORY 3 SCORE: ______ = **TOTAL MOLD RISK** ______

TOTAL MOLD RISK RESULTS

0-4 = **Not Likely Mold Sickness**
5-9 = **Possible Mold Sickness**
10+ = **Probable Mold or Biotoxin Sickness**

OTHER THINGS TO CONSIDER:

- LYME DISEASE, MSIDS, TICK-BORNE COINFECTIONS (USE HORROWITZ MSIDS-LYME QUESTIONNAIRE)
- OTHER ENVIRONMENTAL TOXINS (IE: MERCURY, LEAD, PM2.5, GLYPHOSATE, PESTICIDES, VOCs)
- INTESTINAL PARASITES, CHRONIC VIRAL SYNDROMES, OR OTHER STEALTH INFECTIONS
- FOOD SENSITIVITIES
- CVIDS OR IMMUNODEFICIENCY SYNDROMES

This tool is intended as a clinical information aid, and is not intended to diagnose or treat disease. Symptoms listed have been reported in mold illness patients. Not all symptoms have been proven in studies.

PART 1
DIRTY ROTTEN MOLD

Wish I Had Known

I wish I had known about mold when it really counted.

I missed mold—in my patients, in my family, in myself, and in my own home. I didn't know how to recognize it, and I underestimated the damage it could do.

I wrote this book to myself, 15 years in the past. I needed this book back then. If I would've had it, I may have been able to save patients and loved ones from harm—from months of lost health, life, money, and joy.

I've learned a lot. I've got mold's number now. I want to arm you with what I've learned; with the knowledge and tools you need to conquer the mold in your life. You'll be equipped with proven tools to fight mold and win.

You need mold solutions. This book has them.

WHY YOU'RE READING THIS BOOK

Why else? You want to get better. You want a list of symptoms and cures. Of course. Hey, I'm an impatient learner so I get it. If that's you, flip forward to *Part 2—The 5 Tools*. Check out the solutions.

But then I suggest you spend some time here in *Part 1—Dirty Rotton Mold* to gain a full understanding of mold. Learn what makes it tick and how to truly defeat mold so it never comes back. As one of the oldest living creatures on the planet, mold is an adept survivor. It has a tendency to come back again and again and again. You need to learn its weaknesses to conquer mold for good.

WHY TRUST ME?

I've been there. I've not only worked with mold-sick patients as their doctor, I've been a mold-sick patient myself. I became an expert on mold the hard way, grinding through the day-to-day issues of dealing with the toxic effects of mold. I empathize with you if you're finding this book as a victim of mold sickness yourself.

As a doctor, I worked with a fair number of patients with chronic fatigue and illnesses that nobody could figure out. That's how I came to mold illness. I'm a naturopathic doctor, which means I've been trained to find and treat the cause of "dis-ease." Why is that important? Because usually once the cause of "dis-ease" is removed, people get better. It can be quite elegant and simple. The body has an innate drive to heal. The tricky part is identifying the cause. Sleuthing out the cause is a large part of being a doctor.

Typically, using naturopathic principles to work *with* the body rather than *against* it is pretty effective. But I had this small group of "stuck" patients who didn't respond to the usual things in the usual ways. These patients weren't getting better. Not much changed from appointment to appointment, despite their hard work. Honestly, I was surprised they had enough faith in me to keep coming back.

Then one of those patients found toxic mold in his house—toxic black mold. And I wondered if that might be part of the reason he wasn't getting better despite being 110% dedicated to his treatment plan. I wondered if that might be the reason the others were still sick. I didn't know because I frankly wasn't familiar with all the facets of mold sickness.

I hit the books and was shocked to find that mold was definitely the reason he wasn't responding. The same was true for many of my other "stuck" patients. I was astounded. Even though I found a ton of research on molds, mold toxins, and how they harm living beings, I didn't have a grasp of this in practice. Why? The reason is simple—lack of human studies.

The many research studies about molds and mold toxins (called mycotoxins) are related to animals and animal feed. People in charge of feeding livestock know about the risks. They've even developed mold mitigation techniques to keep their animals healthy.

But there's been little funding to bring this research forward to humans and human impacts. With no definitive lab tests and no vetted treatment protocols from human research, doctors treating real human patients were destined to miss mold just like I did.

Little has changed in the decades since I became aware of mold and mold toxin illness. We now have better lab testing, but still very few human trials to test treatments. Even so, we can learn from the animals because many of the same rules apply to humans as animals. And we can learn from our elders.

Using my knowledge of science, historical treatments, and teachings from mentors, I developed methods to address mold in my "stuck" patients . . . and they improved.

THE ORIGINAL INDOOR ENVIRONMENTAL ILLNESS

I refer to mold illness as "the original indoor environmental illness" because it has been an issue for as long as humans have been inhabiting indoor spaces, from caves to wood huts to stone houses. Mold is even mentioned in the Bible as both a physical body and a spiritual sickness. Even though there are very few human trials on mold treatments, effective treatments have been around for centuries.

Lack of research is not the same as lack of efficacy. Traditional medicine healers from all indigenous cultures successfully treated people afflicted with mold. Sadly, little of that knowledge got passed down to modern day doctors.

Even though I had finally determined mold was the problem for my "stuck" patients, I was left feeling ill equipped without a modern plan or protocol to help them. I had to rely on my teachers, on my scientific training, and a little bit of experimenting.

I studied the animal research to understand how mold hurts living beings. With my comfort in using plants and nutrients, I translated animal research to my understanding of how the human body works. I developed treatments to address the specific problems that mold creates. Incorporating techniques from my teachers, I "practiced" on my mold-sick patients, and had pretty good success. Suddenly, these "stuck" patients followed the script. By removing and treating the cause, they got better.

Since then, I've been on a mission to educate doctors. I created a medical-level mold course teaching about mold sickness in humans. I included the latest in diagnostic tests and treatment. If you want your doctor to become mold-literate, suggest this course series on DrCrista.com: *Doctors—Are you missing mold illness in your patients?* Then, they will also understand the scientific basis for the information in this book.

EARNING MY STRIPES

Mold got to me personally. Ironically, the winter I spent creating the mold course for doctors, mold sprouted in my own home. The entire time I was researching mold illness and creating course material, I was getting sicker and sicker and didn't realize it. I missed the fact that my family and I were sick from mold, even though I was a mold educator. There's a term for this—mold brain. Mold brain is when you simply can't get your brain to work right, like there's a cloud or fog you wish you could shake off.

I underestimated mold. We moved into a relatively new home in late summer. From the time we moved in, as long as it wasn't raining, we kept windows wide open. It was a gorgeous, unseasonably dry autumn, so that meant the windows were open almost all the time. If you haven't spent time in Wisconsin in the fall, I highly recommend it. It's lovely. As winter arrived, we closed up the house more and more, and finally turned on the heat. My children and I started having strange symptoms, but I missed it. I missed mold in my own house.

HOW TO COOK A FROG

Have you heard of the concept of "cooking a frog"? Supposedly, if you put a frog in boiling water, it'll jump out immediately. It senses the drastic, life-threatening change and jumps to safety as quickly as possible. But if you put a frog in cold water and very slowly turn up the heat, it'll stay in the water and eventually boil. Its adaptability is its downfall. Now, I haven't personally tested this theory due to my adoration of amphibians, but I believe this phenomenon was at play in my situation.

As the weather got colder, we closed windows a little more each week. As the fresh, clean outside air decreased, our exposure to sick indoor air increased. This was effectively the same as slowly turning up the heat on the frog. Since it happened slowly, there were no glaring warning signs. My body alarms didn't go off. Our adaptability was our downfall. By slowly being exposed to more and more mold toxins, our frogs got cooked.

Thankfully, our water issue revealed itself on the ceiling in our kitchen. The seam of two drywall pieces started to crack open with a slightly yellow stain. In a few weeks' time, that little yellow stain blossomed into a full-on flood in my kitchen from the bathroom above. Apparently the water made it all the way to my basement and had done so since the house was built. Each of these water-damaged spaces ended up having toxic mold growth, which affected the majority of the rooms in our home.

As you see, I'm coming by this mold sickness stuff honestly. I've personally been knocked down by mold, so have my kids, and so have my patients. When I look back, there are many patients where I think, "Oh my goodness, that was mold sickness. I missed it." Mold sickness might look like sinusitis, asthma, allergies, food sensitivities, chronic skin rashes, anxiety, insomnia, irritable bowel, or an irritable bladder. Mold causes liver disease, kidney disease, and some cancers.

You already know people with mold sickness. Think about the individuals in your life who don't seem to be able to get it together. They may get sick all the time. Or when they do get sick, it takes them a while to kick it. They miss work. They miss school. They make plans but then cancel at the last minute. They have been given strange diagnoses that no one understands, with treatment options that are limited, are risky, or may not work, and with words like idiopathic or sarcoid, start with "pneumo" or end with "itis". Because mold affects many systems in the body, it can look like many other illnesses. Maybe you are that person. Fill out the Crista Mold Questionnaire at the beginning of the book to see if you're displaying mold symptoms. If so, you aren't alone.

I'm very passionate about spreading the word about mold. When the water problem in our house became evident, all of the puzzle pieces came together to reveal that mold was the problem. I instantly began using protocols that I used with my mold-sick patients, in addition to remediation, and we got better. If you're sick from mold, you need the tools in this book.

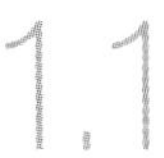

1.1 Hidden Agenda

Mold's hidden agenda is also its purpose on the planet: to recycle and decompose. In fairness, we need mold. We couldn't do without it. Mold transforms plant debris into nutrients for new plant growth. So mold is pretty useful—outside. Not inside. Once it gets a taste of easy living indoors, mold gets out of control. Mold's altruistic purpose skews into a hidden agenda of survival and world domination. If allowed, it will take over your building, your belongings, and your body.

Facts you need to know about mold:

MOLD…

1. is a survivor
2. has bad gas
3. is a bully
4. invades your body
5. causes toxic breath
6. won't go down without a fight
7. turns you into a wimp
8. causes cravings
9. can make you feel crazy, hazy and lazy
10. causes allergies
11. causes food sensitivities
12. makes you sensitive to chemicals
13. makes you sensitive to electromagnetic fields
14. sickness is hard to identify
15. sickness is often misdiagnosed
16. is part of a scandalous cover-up

The next sections elaborate on each point. However, if the bullet-point version is enough for you, skip to section *1.3 Mold Sickness Symptoms* and see if you recognize yourself or someone you know. Either way, keep in mind, if you have mold sickness, you can get better!

1 MOLD IS A SURVIVOR

Mold is the ultimate survivor. It's like the Navy Seal of the fungal world. As one of the oldest living species on earth, it has survival tactics figured out:

- Ⓐ Mold knows how to lurk inside buildings undetected.
- Ⓑ Mold can survive on hidden moisture sources.
- Ⓒ Mold competes for territory by taking out its opponents.
- Ⓓ Mold is tenacious; it'll hunker down and wait out adversity until the coast is clear when it can grow again.

Ⓐ Mold knows how to lurk inside a building undetected. It can grow inside a building without a trace. Mold exists undetected because you often can't see it or smell it. It grows under flooring and behind walls. People often mistake it for dust or carpet stains. Toxic indoor mold rarely has an odor if it's not exposed to air. If you smell a musty, mildewy, or moldy odor, there's definitely a problem. Just know this; mold can be lurking without creating any scent at all.

Ⓑ Mold can survive on hidden moisture sources. Mold only needs a bit of excess humidity to grow. Visible water *is not* required. Mold exists on a microscopic level. An insignificant amount of moisture to us may be like lakefront property to a mold spore. High indoor humidity and dampness is all it takes.

Mold eats any carbohydrate-rich material. It's not picky. Mold will feed on drywall, plywood, subfloor, carpet, cardboard, cork, particleboard, oriented strand board (OSB), or as a carpenter friend calls them, "was-woods." Materials that are broken up or coated in paper are choice food for mold. The more chewed up or broken down it is, the better. That's why OSB grows more mold than plywood—it's just that much more predigested.

Mold can even grow on cement if it's dusty.

Dust **Feeds** Mold

Speaking of dust, it's one of the easiest ways to feed mold. Add high indoor humidity and you've just fed *and* watered mold spores. Think about picture frames, tops of door jams, tops of books on a book shelf, storage items. How often are these typically dusted?

(Side Note: Editors of this book said they paused here to go dust their homes and offices. If you feel compelled to dust, go for it. It's natural. You're not a hypochondriac. You're a life learner and being proactive. The book will be here when you get back. Now get dusting.)

Ⓒ **Mold competes for territory by taking out its opponents.** Mold is a fighter and stealth survivor. If mold has found a sweet spot, it'll fight for it. If other molds or bacteria want to invade its newly found home, mold will emit toxic chemicals to poison the invaders. These chemicals are called mycotoxins.

Ⓓ **Mold is tenacious.** A mold colony will sacrifice resources to ensure survival of the species. If the colony senses a threat, it will shoot spores far into the air with the hopes that its little spore babies will find greener pastures.

I think of mold spores as baby Superman's pod. When Superman's parents knew their planet was going to be destroyed, they loaded their little baby in a pod and shot him out into space, a beacon of hope for the species. This pod was equipped with everything baby Superman would need to sustain life until he found a hospitable new planet. Spores are just like Superman's pod. They're equipped with a bit of food, survival intel, and a mode of delivery to find a new place to land and grow. Spore pods are floating around in the air all the time looking for a bit of moisture.

Don't let your indoor environment become a hospitable planet to mold. Be diligent to control indoor humidity.

2 MOLD HAS BAD GAS

Indoor molds emit many toxic gases, but mycotoxins are the most dangerous. Mycotoxins are poisonous enough to be made into chemical weapons. Weaponized mold toxins are created and stored by militaries around the world. I don't say that to be an alarmist, but rather to make the point of their toxicity. That's how powerful and potentially dangerous mold toxins are. Mold mycotoxins require trained professionals with appropriate protective gear. Now that's some bad gas! Why would we want to live with it in our homes?

Humans and pets get caught in the crossfire when indoor molds compete for territory. Indoor molds fire off gas bombs to kill other mold types. Mold toxins then seep through drywall, insulation, flooring, paint, and many other building materials to pollute our indoor air and our belongings. And you can't detect them by smell.

That's right...mycotoxins, the most poisonous aspect of mold, have no detectable odor.

Mycotoxins Have **No Scent**

But of course we've all smelled mold—that musty, mildewy smell. Those odors are from the other chemicals pumped out by mold, such as volatile organic compounds (VOCs), aldehydes and alcohols. They smell bad when they're exposed to air. If mold is trapped behind building materials, your nose probably won't pick up the scent.

When we walk through a cloud of invisible, odorless mycotoxins, they get into our bodies. Mold mycotoxins can travel much deeper into our lungs than mold spores. They're different from spores. Spores are like pods or seeds, a unit of living material, whereas mycotoxins are a chemical, like a gas.

YOUR LUNGS VERSUS MOLD

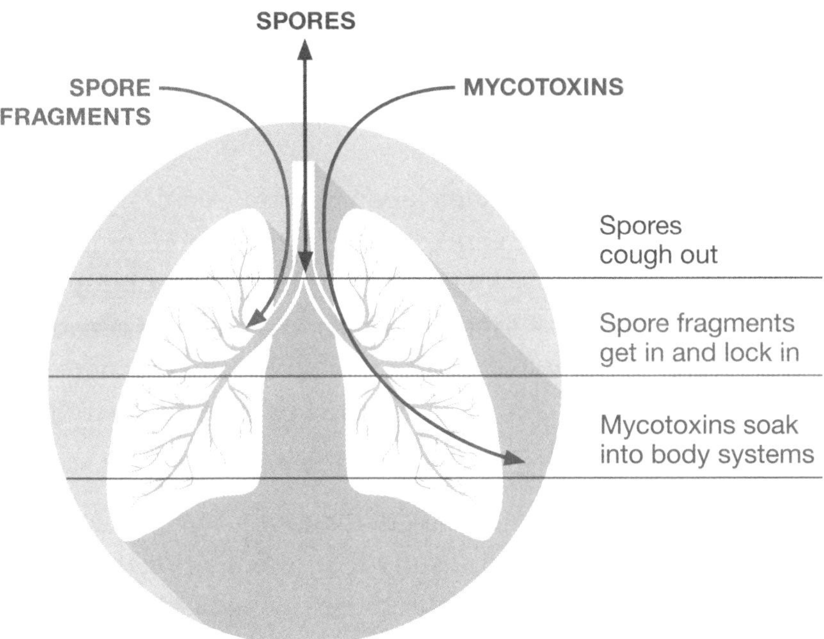

Mycotoxins are 50 times smaller than spores. They can get farther down our respiratory passages and can traverse across the linings of the nose, sinuses and lungs. Our skin has no defense against mycotoxins, especially our hands and feet. And if we eat them, they can wear down the lining of our intestines and move into our vital organs. They can even cross the placenta and affect unborn babies.

Mycotoxins harm all living beings—human, animal, and plant.

If you smell a musty, mildewy, moldy odor, run away. That means mold gases are seeping into your body and affecting your health. Musty odors equal toxic chemicals.

I never imagined that mold could be the problem in my house. Our home wasn't old, and it didn't smell musty. I don't know about you, but I equated mold problems with older homes. I had myself convinced that since I'm very sensitive to mold and didn't smell an odor, the house was fine.

I underestimated the problem.

3 MOLD IS A BULLY

Mold acts like a bully. It picks on certain people more than others. Some people are very sensitive to mold, and some aren't. Mold seems to have a knack for finding susceptible people. This susceptibility has to do with how each of us is genetically wired. It has nothing to do with how physically strong we are. I've seen competitive athletes crippled by mold after trying to do their own mold cleanup without protective gear.

I consider mold sickness a "canary illness." Canary illnesses are caused by environmental insults that affect all of us in large doses, but some of us in small doses. The small-dose sensitive people would be really good canaries in a coal mine. Canaries alert the coal miners that noxious gases are rising to unsafe levels, and that they should get out of the mine.

> Everyone **Reacts** to Mold **Differently**

But remember what happens to the canary? It stops singing because it dies! The canaries get so deeply harmed by the environmental toxin, they keel over. It's a morbid but effective practice to keep the human miners safe. If the miners don't heed the warning from the dead bird, they'll keel over too.

It's the same thing with mold. Mold affects everyone differently. The first to react are the canaries. Mold exploits this sensitivity and can have the rest of the world questioning the validity of their claims. If you have someone in your life "singing like a canary" about feeling sick, and you've had water damage, please listen to them—for your health.

The variance in sensitivity can be explained by genetics. Each individual body with its unique genetics and previous health status will react to toxic mold differently. For instance, some people have allergies to mold spores. Some people don't. Some people are genetically susceptible to mold toxins, and some people aren't. No single body reacts the same as another to the same amount of mold spores or mold toxins. But I guarantee you that no "body" escapes the dangers of mycotoxins. Remember, militaries use them as weapons for a reason. It's simply a matter of dose and duration that makes the difference.

4 MOLD INVADES YOUR BODY

Mold from a sick building can invade your body. If you lived or worked in a moldy environment, you may still be sick even if you've left the sick building. Even though you're no longer being exposed, you may have brought the mold with you on your stuff and inside your body.

Water-damaged buildings create unhealthy ecosystems. They play host to an unruly cast of characters. Like Mad Max, everyone is in it for himself, and others can't be trusted. Life-hackers. Creatures such as fungi, bacteria, and parasites.

They form what's called a biofilm—a slime layer of biological material. This bad-guy slime layer survives in sick environments by cloaking the bad guys and providing a sharing network similar to the dark web. The bad guys share survival code with each other, while competing for who will end up on top. For instance, based on everyone's spies, they decide if the coast is clear to procreate or if it's safe to send out new spores.

The bad guys in the biofilm try to win by poisoning the other players. Think of the vehicles in Mad Max, blowing exhaust gases in the face of the competition. These gases—mycotoxins and bacterial endotoxins—are what make us sick.

> You **Bring the Problem With You** Wherever You Go

The intel from the sick-building biofilm is shared with the critters that have established themselves in your body. The biofilm of that building becomes the biofilm in your body. This may happen in your sinuses, lungs, or digestive system. Just because you left the building, doesn't mean you left the problem behind you.

5 MOLD CAUSES TOXIC BREATH

When mold invades your body, it inhabits your sinuses primarily. Mold gives you bad breath, but not in the way you might be thinking. It's not stinky breath, it's more like toxic breath, meaning toxin-carrying breath. Because sinus molds from water-damaged buildings exist in a competitive biofilm, they're actively spitting out mycotoxins to poison any other critter that wants to infringe on their territory.

This makes your breath toxic—to yourself and to others. Every time you inhale, you breathe in mold mycotoxins. Every time you exhale, you breathe out mold mycotoxins. Inhaled mycotoxins absorb into your body. Exhaled mycotoxins can make those close to you sick. In my medical practice, family members of mold-sick patients often developed mold symptoms even though their mycotoxin tests were clear.

Some people dispute the idea that sinus mold is a problem. If we were to scope up inside everyone's noses, we'd see that all of us have a little mold fungi in our sinuses. So if everyone has fungus up there, why do some people get sick and some people don't?

The reason? Exposure to a water-damaged building makes all the difference.

> **Water-Damaged Building Exposure is the Key** That Turns Normal Sinus Fungus Into Bad-Guy Fungus

Researchers refer to this as colonization because it's not really an infection. Once your nasal fungi are exposed to the unhealthy ecosystem of a water-damaged building, they turn criminal. A colony once peacefully coexisting turns into an apocalyptic landscape.

6 MOLD WON'T GO DOWN WITHOUT A FIGHT

As mold dies, it goes down with guns a'blazin. Dying mold spits out more mycotoxins than living mold. And if that wasn't bad enough, each mycotoxin is made more toxic in the presence of any other mycotoxin. It's called an additive effect. In a typical water-damaged building, there's more than one mold species trying to establish dominance. Remember Mad Max. With weapons drawn, dying colonies of bad-guy biofilm will gas bomb the whole environment. I picture mold saying, "if I'm going down, I'm taking you with me."

At certain concentrations, a building's contents will actually accumulate mycotoxins—only to be off-gassed later over time. This is why some people don't get better after mold remediation. Mycotoxins are left in the building's materials.

Another problem with dying mold is that it breaks into small fragments. Fragments are formed at an alarming rate. A single spore can break into 500 fragments. Fragments are smaller than spores but not as small as mycotoxins. As shown in the lung diagram, fragments can travel farther into the lungs, past the lung's clearing defense system. They sit there, perpetually irritating the lung tissue. The fragments carry DNA protein pieces that trigger allergic reactions.

Because of mycotoxin increase and fragment formation, I commonly recommend that people avoid do-it-yourself (DIY) cleanups, especially if already having symptoms. It's not worth it. Call the professionals.

7 MOLD TURNS YOU INTO A WIMP

Mold weakens immune defenses in a few different ways. Mycotoxins reduce the immune system's ability to fight infections. You might find that you get sick more often. Or, when you do get sick, you can't seem to kick it like you used to. Mold-sick people often say that colds go on forever or always go to their sinuses. It's common to see asthma flare.

If you're really immune impaired from mold, you may not be able to get a cold at all. Mold can rewire the immune system at the genetic level. With this new wiring, people don't get classically sick, but they feel low-grade terrible all the time without knowing why. Viral infections go chronic and fly under the radar of detection from doctors.

The immune system is not only in charge of fighting infection but also in cleaning up garbage in the body. People with mycotoxin poisoning get sluggish from excess waste in their bodies. That's one of the ways mold increases the risk for some cancers.

We feel too cruddy to get out. We stay in the environment, and eventually mycotoxins build to cancer-causing levels. Toxic mold is especially carcinogenic to those with chronic viral infections—an unfair double-whammy.

8 MOLD CAUSES CRAVINGS

Earlier I mentioned that mold only needs a tiny bit of carbohydrate to survive. So what do you think people with mold colonies in their sinuses crave? Carbohydrates! The simpler the carb, the better. I'm talking pasta, breads, cookies, crackers, muffins, cereal, and anything made with flour. But mold really would prefer that you go straight for the sugar: sugar in your coffee, brown sugar in your oatmeal, and candy. The sugars in alcohol are its favorites.

Mold Makes You **Crave Sugar**

If mold is not fed, it begins to die inside your body. As it dies, mold releases toxic chemicals that travel to your brain and affect how you think. Without sweets, mold-sick people describe a sense of deep fog over the brain. Like Tom Hanks' character in Joe Versus the Volcano who's diagnosed with a "brain cloud."

These chemicals also increase pain all over the body. No wonder people eat sweets! It's better than feeling cloudy and in pain. Or, you could treat your mold sickness.

As discussed, mold colonizes in the sinuses, but small amounts can also migrate to lungs and intestines. In some people, especially those on long-term steroid medications, mold in the gut becomes a dense biofilm. The biofilm hosts a gut fungus called candida which gobbles up the food for itself and reduces nutrient absorption through the intestinal lining. We see odd cravings in these mold sufferers as they try to get enough nutrients.

9 MOLD CAN MAKE YOU FEEL CRAZY, HAZY & LAZY

Mold sufferers are often misunderstood. They can start to feel a little crazy. If they're canaries, they may start to feel sick before others around them. The symptoms they feel are very real physical symptoms. But mold symptoms are vague, show up in many different areas, and may be easily explained away as something else.

Mold affects each person differently. It often isn't obvious that mold is the problem because it's hidden. So, mold-sick people feel like hypochondriacs. They look around wondering if other people are feeling the same way. Take heart canaries, you aren't crazy. A simple medical test can confirm your sanity. See section *1.4 Diagnostics & Tests*.

I use the word hazy to describe the cognitive difficulties and vision changes I've observed in my mold-sick patients. Many say it's like feeling a little buzzed or slightly drunk. They simply can't get their brains to work right. Vision is often affected, causing blurring. Some report issues focusing, as if the left and right eyes are no longer coordinated. These vision changes can come and go, so people blame it on being tired.

People with mold sickness often complain of feeling tired—not sleepy tired—more like fatigue or feeling worn out. Some describe it as running on "low battery." Sometimes they perk up when they get out of the sick environment, but not necessarily. It's not that easy. Mold-sick people have bad-actor mold in their sinuses and bring the problem with them wherever they go. Researchers have found a high correlation between people with chronic fatigue syndrome and people who've been exposed to water-damaged buildings. It isn't laziness; it's illness.

10 MOLD CAUSES ALLERGIES

If you've been exposed to a water-damaged building, you can develop allergies…to anything. Of course you can develop an allergy to mold, but also pollen, grass, dust, pet dander, and so on. You name it, you can develop an allergy to it. One person

I worked with developed an allergy to grapes, so you never know.

Mold causes allergic reactions to anything you're exposed to on a regular basis. In the Mold Turns You Into A Wimp section, I talk about how mold can rewire your immune system. Not only does the rewiring make your immune system wimpy to viruses, it also causes your system to overreact in inappropriate ways. Pollen is not out to get you, but it can sure feel that way if you have an allergy to it. Allergic reactions are miserable and debilitating.

Here's a hint that an allergy could actually be mold at the core. If a normally healthy person has either moved or taken a new job, and the next season develops a new allergy, think mold. Quite often, when mold is addressed, these allergies go away.

11 MOLD CAUSES FOOD SENSITIVITIES

If you're being exposed to mold, you can develop food sensitivities. Just like in the previous section, you can develop allergic reactions to anything you eat on a regular basis. Under the influence of mold, your body begins to view commonly eaten foods as a perpetual threat, something to be attacked. This can cause bloating and inflammation in the intestines.

Mycotoxins can be ingested in the food we eat. This is true for pets as well. Mycotoxins are most often found in grains, flour, and dried fruit. Mold may be a contributor to the growing trend of grain allergies. When mycotoxins travel down the digestive tract, they destroy the intestinal lining. Our smart bodies try to get rid of the toxins by flushing the colon, causing diarrhea. Then constipation may follow. It's not unusual for mold-sick people to develop irritable bowels, alternating constipation with diarrhea, or as one of my patients describes it, "consti-rrhea."

12 MOLD MAKES YOU SENSITIVE TO CHEMICALS

Mycotoxins are toxic chemicals that need to be removed from the body as safely as possible. We rely on our liver and kidneys to do this job. These organs make mycotoxins less dangerous by packaging them to be dumped in stool and urine.

Unfortunately, mold makes far more mycotoxins than our bodies can handle. A 1-inch square of mold contains more than 1 million spores. All day long, day after day, mold pumps out toxic gases. This equates to many balloons full of poisonous gas for our liver and kidneys to manage. They can't keep up, and they get backlogged.

Backlogged organs can't do their normal job of processing all the other chemicals we encounter every day. Chemicals found in perfumes, cleaning products, personal care products, and candles become hard to handle. It's very common for a mold-sick person to gravitate toward unscented and natural products.

13 MOLD MAKES YOU SENSITIVE TO ELECTROMAGNETIC FIELDS

At the cellular level, mold changes our sensitivity to electrical currents. Electromagnetic fields (EMFs), such as Wi-Fi, do the same. Mold-sick people have a harder time being around EMFs because mold has impaired their sensitivity to electrical signals. This is an oversimplification of the science, but I wanted to comment on this commonly seen but rarely studied phenomenon.

We actually make "good" EMFs inside our body when we move our skeletal system and muscles—in other words, when we exercise. Even though these EMFs are "good," they don't feel good to a sensitized person. People exposed to water-damaged buildings tend to move less and less to reduce the EMF burden.

There's that lazy thing again. Mold would be perfectly happy to have you lay around long enough for it to compost you. Yikes! Make sure to fight it and keep moving.

14 MOLD SICKNESS IS HARD TO IDENTIFY

Most people develop mold sickness slowly over the course of a few months. Their symptoms are vague, low grade, and likely different from others with the same exposure. Because mold can hide inside a building, the symptoms aren't often tied back to mold. One clue it might be mold is if symptoms are worse on rainy days, after snow melt, with barometric pressure changes, and after eating carbs.

Mold is difficult to identify even for trained medical practitioners. It was for me. I needed a clinical tool. That's why I developed the Crista Mold Questionnaire. It can be filled out on your own and given to your doctor. Use it to get an idea if mold might be an issue for you, and then again throughout your treatment to track progress. Check all the boxes that apply to you, and tally your score.

15 MOLD SICKNESS IS OFTEN MISDIAGNOSED

Mold is misunderstood by the conventional medical community. The conversation on mold illness stops at "spore sickness." By "spore sickness," I'm referring to symptoms caused by a direct reaction to mold spores. This is often called a mold allergy.

Mold allergy is a thing, but it's only a single aspect of a more complicated picture. Mold mycotoxins are a much bigger problem, and more damaging. When I think of mold sickness, I include both "spore" and "mycotoxin" illnesses.

Spores can irritate the eyes, nose, throat, sinuses, inner ear, and lungs, whereas mycotoxins disperse far and wide. They can enter the body if we breathe them, eat them, and absorb them through our skin. Mycotoxins harm the entire respiratory tract, eyes, ears, intestines, liver, kidneys, skin, nerves, immune system, bone marrow, bladder, and brain. With that many areas, it's difficult to pinpoint one symptom as mold sickness.

Spore Symptoms + Mycotoxin Symptoms
= **Mold Sickness**

Don't be upset if your doctor hasn't discussed mold sickness with you yet. Your doctor wants to help you. That's why s/he became a doctor. It's not from a lack of caring but from a lack of awareness of mold's potential to create harm. I've given professional-level education courses to doctors of all types. Many are thankful for being made aware of the problem and want to learn possible solutions, whether or not they have a comfort level using natural medicines. Doctors want to help their patients.

I think the main difficulty has been a lack of generally accepted laboratory testing. It has been difficult to prove exposure to the toxic aspects of mold: the mycotoxins, alcohols, aldehydes, and VOCs. Now that testing is improving, I hope the medical community can move forward in their understanding and catch mold when it's the issue.

16 MOLD IS PART OF A SCANDALOUS COVER-UP

Here's the deal, mold sickness is rampant and unrecognized. The Occupational Safety and Health Association (OSHA) estimates that 1 out of 4 buildings has had enough water damage to grow toxic mold, molds that negatively affect human health. That's a ton of people at risk.

Unfortunately, there are parties interested in suppressing information about mold sickness. Many mold stories start with a horror story about college housing, living in a basement, summer camp, volunteering, or being the new guy at work assigned the nasty cleanup job.

Many mold stories also involve someone who knew there was a mold problem, was dishonest, and hid the problem. Entities that stand to lose money are insurance companies, landlords, companies where there's occupational exposure, and homeowners in cahoots with real estate agents. Don't be fooled; this is absolutely about money.

For instance, I recently stayed at a very nice resort for a conference. People at the conference started seeking me out because of symptoms they developed in a certain conference room: brain fog, confusion, sleepiness, runny nose, sore throat, post-nasal drip, and heart palpitations to name a few. Conferences are expensive, so they were trying to tough it out to get the information they paid for. Eventually, management was called and I was brought in as the mold expert.

When I stepped into the room, I could tell there was a problem. My ears started ringing immediately. I noticed a moldy area on the ceiling from a roof leak. It was clearly water-damaged, with rotting wood, and was covered in a fine white dust. When I pointed it out, management said it wasn't mold, just dust. I asked for the test as proof because there's no way to visually diagnose mold. Scientific sampling and diagnostic tests must be done.

Those tests hadn't been done. I was told that maintenance asked an expert who said it wasn't the bad kind of mold, so they left it. They made a decision to save money and ignore the problem.

Incidentally, the conference organizers listened to their attendees and moved to a new location. Rather than remove the material, the resort brushed off the problem to save money. Did that really work in the end?

> Indoor Mold is **Never Okay**—Ever, Ever, Ever

Any mold and any mildew indoors is bad news! Some are worse than others, but all have bad gas. Yes that includes mildew. Mildew is in the mold family. It isn't in the family of the toxic indoor molds, but mildew still secretes many of the same chemicals, such as VOCs. That's no good in the air you breathe.

1.2

Know Your Foe

The drywall seam that came apart in my kitchen ceiling had apparently been there for weeks. I didn't notice it. My family did and figured I saw it. In those few weeks, a gazillion mold spores aggressively grew behind the drywall, between the shower above and the ceiling below. Mold can grow on a moist surface in 24 to 48 hours. Of course, it's best to be vigilant and react quickly to any water problem, but what if you don't notice it?

Here are the most common molds and mycotoxins you'll find in an indoor environment. The one that gets all the press is "black mold" or Stachybotrys, but all mycotoxins harm human health. You don't have to know this to get better. There's no test. This is for the nerds who think it's neat. And it might help you connect the dots when you test your body.

MYCOTOXIN	MOLD SOURCE
Aflatoxin	Aspergillus flavus Aspergillus parasiticus
Chaetoglobosin A	Chaetomium globosum
Enniatin B	Fusarium species
Gliotoxin	Aspergillus fumigatus
Ochratoxin A	Aspergillus ochraseus Aspergillus niger Penicillium verrucosum Penicillium nordicum Penicillium chrysogenum
Roridin E	Stachybotrys chartarum Fusarium species
Sterigmatocystin	Aspergillus versicolor
Verrucarin A	Stachybotrys chartarum Fusarium species
Zearalenone	Fusarium species

Remember, indoor molds also spit out other chemicals such as VOCs, aldehydes, and alcohols.

TALES AS MOLD AS TIME

I don't know about you, but I remember stories much easier than tables and bullet-point lists, so I made sure to sprinkle in a few, in case you learn like I do. In these stories, you might notice that there isn't one consistent picture of mold sickness. It can look different in each person and cause many kinds of symptoms.

You may also notice that most of the people in the stories had other diagnoses that could have explained away the symptoms. You may also notice that the hero in each story showed improvement by treating mold, and showed the most improvement by getting away from the moldy environment. Hearing other people's stories makes it interesting and brings hope. If you're dealing with mold sickness, I hope one of these stories fuels your drive to get better.

It's story time!

STORY | **THE MYSTERIOUS CASE OF THE INJURED HOCKEY PLAYER**

The mother of a hockey family brought in her teen son for help with a stinger—a painful pinched nerve in the neck. It wouldn't go away and was ruining his prospects for a career in hockey. Scouts were looking at him for college, but the stinger had developed into crippling nerve pain down his shooting arm. It started after an illegal check. After the hit, he had persistent ear ringing. Teammates teased that he got his bell rung.

Physical therapy put him on forced rest and gave him exercises. Things improved, but would worsen once he got back to practice. He saw a highly skilled team of practitioners—neurologist, rheumatologist, physical therapist, chiropractor, massage therapist, and, finally psychiatrist, in case it was all in his head. Nothing seemed to help. He got worse every time he went back to practice. This poor kid tried everything—special diets, exercises, counseling, yet the stinger wouldn't go away. He wanted to get better and play hockey, but he was running short on luck.

When I did a full review of his symptoms, I learned more information. He mentioned being annoyed by how often he had to come off the ice to pee. It was only an issue when he was skating. He also mentioned foul-smelling gas and sweet cravings. He had a long history of sciatica from skating that acted up at practice, but he learned to live with it. He also had rashes wherever his pads touched his skin, and itchy athlete's foot. But he said, "all hockey players have skin stuff."

Whenever I see urinary frequency along with ear ringing, nerve pains, and skin rashes, mold is on my list of possible considerations. Add athlete's foot, sweet cravings, and gas, and mold rises in my suspicion.

We did some investigating into his environment and found that mold was growing in his locker at the rink. His pads, his skates, and his helmet were moldy. They were handed down from brother to brother, and they all joked that they smelled "rank." They never connected the smell with harmful mycotoxins. His equipment was stored in the locker room; a warm, humid environment with a constant source of moisture from the showers and sweat.

He practiced three hours every day with moldy equipment. He was breathing mycotoxins, and they were soaking through his skin. He was giving himself mold toxicity as he played. When he was on forced rest, his mycotoxin load reduced, and symptoms improved. The kids with lockers next to his weren't as affected because they weren't as genetically susceptible.

Suddenly, with new equipment and a remediation of the locker room, his treatments stuck. The stinger healed for good, ear ringing went away, and sciatica improved. Skin rashes cleared up. He no longer had to urinate as much because his body wasn't being poisoned as he played. Interestingly, not only did his nerve problems get better, his vision also improved. He hadn't noticed it was bad until it got better. ✹

So, was this kid just a wimp? Was he unlucky? Were there unresolved emotional issues about playing hockey that he needed to address through counseling? No. It was mold. When there are real physical impacts on a body that we don't understand, we often shift the blame to something else. Continuing to investigate is more useful to the person who is suffering.

1.3

Mold Sickness Symptoms

Let's talk symptoms. Remember, mold has two types of weapons—spores and gases—the worst of which are mycotoxins. Mold causes symptoms in many areas of the body. Every individual, every unique body chemistry, is affected by mold differently. Some people are extremely sensitive, and some people aren't. Ultimately, it comes down to the total amount of exposure and personal sensitivity.

SYMPTOMS of mold exposure are... wide-reaching
can be vague
rarely exist alone

Mold symptoms don't fit into a tidy checklist that applies to all people. It works better to look at a summation of symptoms. The more mold symptoms we check off, the more confidence we have in the diagnosis of mold sickness.

That said, almost every person with mold sickness I've seen had some level of anxiousness. People around them don't necessarily know it's going on because the mold-sick person deals with it internally.

> There's **No Single Symptom** That Confirms Mold Sickness

It may seem like an internal experience of feeling unsettled, uneasy, overwhelmed, or stressed out. Some describe feeling restless or not being able to find inner stillness or a feeling of impending doom or worrying something bad is going to happen. Others describe dreading social encounters. These feelings improved after the mold was addressed.

STORY | **STRESSED OUT**

A woman came to see me with chronic fatigue syndrome. She was struggling with fatigue, sinus congestion, insomnia and episodes of an unnerving feeling of dread. She used a steroidal sinus spray for the congestion and Tylenol PM to sleep at night. The moments of dread were diagnosed as panic attacks, and they were happening more frequently. She was given antianxiety medication and told to work on managing her stress. Ironically, the medication made her feel more nervous and wiped her out the next day. She wanted to explore other options.

She worked in historic preservation out of a beautifully restored Victorian mansion. For enjoyment, she toured the country visiting historic sites and staying in historic bed and breakfasts. History was her passion. She felt "high-strung" at work, yet noted that she enjoyed calm weekends at home. She believed her chronic fatigue made her feel more stressed at work as she tried to keep up with the pace. The dread feeling was happening more often, and she worried she might have to retire early.

It turns out, the problem was indeed her job, but not the stress of it—rather the environments. We narrowed it down that the feeling of dread was most severe when she was at work and when sleeping in musty rooms while traveling. She worked in a musty space and had "gotten used to it." She thought she developed allergies with age, and was easily stressed out. She didn't connect the dots that mold exposure at work caused her sinus issues and her panic attacks because neither happened immediately after starting to work there.

The building where she worked had an invisible mold problem. It sustained various events of water damage through the years. Her sinus spray contained steroids that helped her breathe, but at a cost. Steroids reduced her immune system's ability to fend off mold spores from the building that wanted to invade her sinuses. Her tests showed multiple strains of mold in her sinuses and a high mycotoxin burden. Her panic attacks were due to mold, not an inability to handle stress.

She moved locations for work and was treated for mold. Not only did the panic attacks go away, she started to sleep better, and she was able to stop using the steroid sinus spray and sleep aid over time. Her fatigue improved. We could've blamed many of her symptoms on stress, but she didn't have to change anything in her life other than her exposures. Not only is she handling work better, she's enjoying it again. ✺

HOW LONG UNTIL SYMPTOMS SHOW UP?

It really varies how long it takes for mold symptoms to show up. Because of differences in individual susceptibilities, mold symptoms can arise anywhere from immediately to months out. They often start quietly—mild and tolerable. It can take months before symptoms are strong enough to be noticed. A typical time frame is 3-6 months.

Women generally have symptoms sooner than men. There's a chemical reason for that. Mycotoxins are fat-soluble, which means they're stored in fat. Like it or not, women tend to have higher body-fat percentages than men. Their burden of fat-soluble toxins can get higher faster. The spillover of these toxins causes symptoms.

EVERY BREATH YOU TAKE

When you're in a water-damaged building or hosting bad-guy biofilm in your sinuses, every breath you take can be harmful. Mold mycotoxins pollute the air. As you breathe, you take on mycotoxins.

For the science nerds, here's a general list of the ways mycotoxins affect living beings:

- Causes inflammation in sinuses, lungs, bladder, and digestive tract
- Migrates across linings of the respiratory and digestive tracts
- Absorbs and stores in fat
- Interferes with vital cellular processes
- Causes mitochondrial damage
- Impairs synthesis of protein, RNA, and DNA
- Depletes the master cell antioxidant called glutathione
- Accelerates programmed cell death
- Is poisonous to nerves in the body and brain
- Is toxic to liver and kidneys
- Affects medications metabolized by the cytochrome p450 system
- Inhibits immune defenses
- Causes some cancers
- Winnows away the lining of the intestines
- Crosses into the brain and weakens the blood-brain barrier
- Rides the olfactory nerve to the hippocampus and frontal lobe
- Crosses the placenta and becomes more active inside the uterus
- Is detectable in breast milk

JUST GIVE ME A LIST

I wish I could give you a list with all the mold symptoms, but that's impossible. There simply isn't enough human research on mold sickness. The lists I provide aren't definitive lists of mold sickness symptoms. I've included some of the most common symptoms seen by mold-literate doctors, as well as those that are highly linked to mold exposure.

Having one symptom from any of these lists doesn't mean you

have mold sickness. If mold is bothering your body, it generally causes more than one symptom in more than one area of your body. To get a better idea if you might have mold sickness, use the Crista Mold Questionnaire at the beginning of the book. Here they are by category.

SYMPTOMS

EYES, EARS, NOSE & THROAT (EENT)

- Sneezing
- Runny nose
- Post-nasal drip
- Chronic sinusitis
- Nasal polyps
- Bumps at back of the throat
- Swollen lymph nodes
- Allergies
- Hay fever
- Ear popping
- Ringing in the ears
- Hearing loss
- Dry eyes
- Irritated eyes

STORY | HAY FEVER

This man's story is typical of mold sickness. He and some buddies finished his basement for a home office. He was a healthy guy who spent a fair amount of time at the gym. Not long after finishing his basement, he developed an allergy to grass pollen. His doctor said that people can develop allergies with aging. He started allergy medication as recommended. Soon after, he developed a sore throat, post-nasal drip, dry irritated eyes, and ear ringing, followed by irritable bowels that didn't seem connected to what he ate.

He started to have trouble focusing on work and felt like taking a nap rather than exercising. He felt much better after exercise, so he forced himself to go. His hay fever progressed from grass season to any season when it wasn't frozen outdoors. Allergy medication was starting to fail him. He developed a faint wheeze when exercising in the cold. His doctor started talking about asthma medication. That's when he came to see me for help.

It turns out that there were errors in his basement buildout that encouraged mold growth. Mold was growing a few inches up from the base of all outside walls—exactly where his corner office was. When the carpet was pulled, the carpet beneath his filing cabinet was moldy as well. Grass wasn't the primary cause. Mold was. The allergies and problems that followed were due to mold's effect on his body. After remediation and treatment, he returned to his old self, but it took longer than he had hoped. We suspected that he was still being exposed to leftover mycotoxins. ❋

SYMPTOMS

RESPIRATORY SYSTEM

- Shortness of breath
- Wheezing
- Asthma
- Chronic dry cough
- Burning lungs
- Heaviness in the chest
- Sensitivity to fragrances
- Colds go to the lungs easily
- Chronic respiratory illnesses
- Blood-stained spit or sputum
- Smoke & exhaust sensitivity
- Aspergillosis

STORY | **THE STUDENT ATHLETE**

One young man I worked with was a college athlete. His complaint was frequent colds that would linger and eventually become bacterial. He was getting colds much more often, which would go to his sinuses or lungs and require antibiotics to clear. Getting sick was affecting his ability to compete.

He had other annoyances that he tolerated, such as insomnia, itchy ears, and "blowing his throat" every morning. He rarely had to blow his nose, even though he had a nasal voice. He had post-nasal drip which cleared up when he went home, but came back when he returned to school.

It turns out he lived in a moldy apartment.

Obviously he didn't have the genetics of an extremely mold-sensitive person. His score on the Crista Mold Questionnaire was only slightly probable for mold. I'm certain that his exercise routine also helped him clear mycotoxins. Living in a moldy environment reduced his ability to fight respiratory viruses and made him more susceptible to bacterial infections.

When we treated the mold, his immune system strengthened, the post-nasal drip halted, he slept better, and he wasn't itching his ears all the time. Best of all, he was a competitor again. When he left the moldy place to take a new job, he thrived. ✹

SYMPTOMS

DIGESTIVE SYSTEM

- Appetite changes
- Nausea
- Irritable bowels
- Diarrhea/Constipation
- Vomiting
- Cyclical vomiting syndrome
- Bloating
- Abdominal pain
- Ulcers
- Food sensitivities
- Sweet cravings

STORY | **COOK'S DILEMMA**

A vegetarian woman in her thirties came for help with an increasingly unpredictable digestive system. A true foodie, she loved eating, cooking, and taking cooking classes. Over the past few years, eating was starting to feel like walking in a minefield, never knowing what was going to land her in the bathroom. Her tipping point was losing wine. She loved wine. She drank wine while cooking, while reading, and with friends. She joined a wine club and was especially good at food and wine pairings. But lately, it was giving her headaches and heartburn.

She felt queasy most of the time with general stomach pain that wasn't necessarily related to eating. Her digestion was starting to rule her life, with events of urgent diarrhea, alternating with uncomfortable gassy constipation. On review, she was also dealing with tingling feet, which she blamed on poor circulation and gaining weight. Her skin was getting more sensitive and breaking out with certain lotions. In the appointment, she seemed easily confused.

She had been tested up and down with only a few vague findings. Upper endoscopy showed esophagitis. The colonoscopy report mentioned degradation of the intestinal lining without ulceration. Celiac and B12 tests were normal. She was diagnosed with irritable bowel syndrome and leaky gut. Medication was offered, but she refused because she feared the side effects.

She wasn't able to pinpoint which foods were causing the problem. In desperation, she tried an elimination-challenge diet, taking out almost all foods, which was a hardship she couldn't maintain. She started having fantasies about pasta and wine. It's not uncommon to crave what we're sensitive to. I asked her to avoid grains and wine, and nothing else. Mean doctor, I know.

She felt much, much better, but because her social life involved food and drink, avoiding her favorite things made her feel isolated. After an intestinal rebuilding phase, we agreed she could try to reintroduce grains, one at a time, very slowly...and then wine. The findings were interesting. She only had a problem with nonorganic grains, and organic (yes, organic) wines. I didn't have any idea what was going on.

Then someone gave a presentation at her wine club about ochratoxin in wine from moldy grapes. Grapes not sprayed by chemical fungi cides are prone to mold growth. Apparently, this is a dirty little secret in the wine industry. This company was one of the few organic wineries that certified its organic wine as free of ochratoxin. The wine guy cracked the code and solved the case. Mold exposure was at the heart of her problems.

The woman connected the timing of her weight gain and digestive problems to when she took a new job. The building where she worked had a leaky ceiling that everyone joked about; even requiring them to use waste baskets to catch water during heavy storms. It was funny. No one thought it might be making them sick because there wasn't any mold to be seen. And besides, she got diarrhea from food, not her building—or so she thought. She was actually getting sick from both. ✹

SYMPTOMS
CIRCULATORY SYSTEM

- Many spider veins
- Cherry angiomas
- Easy bruising
- Easy bleeding
- Iron-deficiency anemia
- Varicose veins
- Raynaud's phenomenon
- Irregular heartbeat
- Low or reactive blood pressure
- Atriovenous malformation

SYMPTOMS
SKIN

- Sensitive skin
- Itchy skin
- Burning sensation
- Flushing
- Sensitivity to sunlight
- Skin rash
- Peeling or sloughing skin
- Fungal infections

STORY | INFANT WITH ECZEMA

The mother of an infant boy sought my help. He was covered with eczema from head to toe. He was so agitated, he couldn't sleep. In the appointment, he whimpered and was clearly miserable. The only thing that kept his tender, irritated skin from cracking was cream containing steroids and antifungal medication. If they missed one dose, he would break out to the point that his skin would crack and bleed.

Feeling helpless, mom turned to the Internet. She read that other nursing moms noticed improvement with diet changes. She was a very proactive and educated mom. Her devotion to him was unending. She worked for three years to get pregnant. As a parent of another child, a four year old with autism, she understood sacrifice for a child.

She watched her baby son's reactions carefully and omitted foods that seemed to make things worse. She was down to lamb, rice, homemade organic bone broth, blueberries, and microgreens.

Other than the antifungal steroid cream, she put nothing on his skin. His clothes were washed in vinegar with an extra rinse, and diapers were organic cotton. There was little I could suggest to improve on this. We added a bath soak of calendula and chamomile tea, which soothed him enough to sleep. I recommended we test his stool for intestinal flora and conduct a full environmental assessment. These proactive parents hired a certified building biologist to check out their lakeside cottage home.

The indoor air inspector called aghast. There was black mold all over this cottage. It was behind the drywall of almost every wall in the house. The humidity was out of control because the house was essentially built on a bog by a lake. The inspector said the builder should never have been granted a building permit on that land.

The baby's stool test came back with excessive yeast overgrowth. He had fungus inside and out. With an autistic sibling, he likely had an inherited genetic susceptibility to environmental toxins. It turns out that everyone in the family was sick in their own way. They went to a hotel while remediation occurred and the little boy's skin cleared up.

Unfortunately in this case, the remediation had to be redone two more times to completely eradicate the mold. Each time they tried to come home, the baby would break out. Thankfully, the parents paid attention. ✺

SYMPTOMS

BRAIN

- Brain fog
- Confusion
- Slowed thinking
- Memory loss
- Trouble finding the right word
- Dementia

STORY | MOLD ON THE MIND

A previously healthy woman in her mid-50s came to see me for help after recently developing muscle twitches. She also had slow, foggy thinking, insomnia, and weak, easily fatigued muscles. She was generally in pretty bad shape and was scared.

During her physical examination, I noted that she had symptoms of an upper motor neuron lesion. This means that based on an individual's muscle weaknesses and twitches, we can determine if the source is the brain. In her case, it was.

She and her husband had built their dream home, a log home in the country. Over the next five years, she had developed insomnia, anxiety, fatigue, and feeling like she was going to die. The muscle twitches were sometimes so severe, they would wake her from sleep. After a lot of diagnostic work, we discovered it was mold toxicity. Her symptoms started right after moving keepsakes from her mother's basement. She brought them to her home for sorting because her mother's house smelled terribly musty and made her feel strange.

She unwittingly infected her pristine home.

The home was remediated and she started treatment. Her mother's moldy belongings were removed, and she temporarily moved to one of her adult children's homes. Despite a comprehensive plan, she couldn't move home for a very long time.

Back then, I wasn't aware of sinus colonies or mycotoxins. I thought mold spores were the whole issue. Now, in retrospect, she probably needed sinus treatment. And if we had rid her body, brain, and belongings of mycotoxins, she may have been able to move home sooner. Instead she required extra time for her brain to rebuild the injured areas to stop the twitching. ✹

SYMPTOMS
NERVOUS SYSTEM

- Anxiousness
- Depression
- Incoordination
- Headache
- Dizziness/Vertigo
- Migraine
- Slow reflexes
- Dysautonomia
- Insomnia
- Neuropathies
- Tremors
- Seizures
- Daytime sleepiness
- Difficulty with balance and walking

STORY | **TREMOR**

A woman in her early 40s came to see me with her husband. She had a recent diagnosis of essential tremor, a condition similar to Parkinson's Disease. Prospects of recovery were not good. Her tremor was constant, affecting her balance and ability to sleep. She had heart palpitations that made her catch her breath. She also constantly felt like she had a bladder infection, even though no infection was found. The urinary frequency was so bad, she had to leave the appointment to urinate. Family said she'd become more weepy, which everyone understood considering her health issues.

Her husband seemed overly anxious about her health. While she was visiting the bathroom, he confided that he felt like he was getting more and more impatient and short with her. His sleep was interrupted with worry. This level of irritability didn't fit the kind and empathetic man in front of me.

On review, she had a tick bite about a year prior to the beginning of her first tremor. The tick was found, removed intact, and sent for testing. It was a Lyme-carrying tick. Even though many people who contract Lyme don't get a rash, she developed a growing red rash where the tick was. It was clear that she needed treatment for Lyme disease. She was given the standard of care at the time, which was later found to be insufficient at eradicating the bacteria.

It was evident to me that the Lyme bacteria might be persisting and affecting her nervous system. The tremor began in her hand on the same side as the tick bite. We started her on a chronic Lyme protocol. She only had minimal improvement. We tried a few tweaks, and still there wasn't much improvement with her tremor. I consulted with Lyme-literate colleagues to check my protocol or to spur ideas, and one mentioned checking into mold.

When I brought this idea up to the couple, the expressions on their faces looked as if I had just found them guilty of a crime. They had water damage in their home and with all that was going on with the wife's Lyme disease, they hadn't addressed it. They closed the door to the wet, musty basement to deal with it later. As mold expert Dr. Sandeep Gupta says, "If there's any part of you that you aren't addressing, eventually it will address you." ❋

SYMPTOMS

URINARY SYSTEM

- Overactive bladder
- Irritable bladder
- Kidney inflammation
- Blood in urine
- Bladder infection symptoms with no identifiable infection

STORY | **KIDNEY DISEASE**

This young man of 21 was living at home with his parents and one sibling. He came to see me for deep-seated fatigue, low-back pain, blood in his urine, and some libido challenges. I hadn't seen him in more than five years. I was struck by his appearance. He looked washed out with very dark circles under his eyes. He wasn't just pale, he was vampire pale.

Dark circles were a clue that he was depleting his health by not getting enough rest, exercise, hydration, or healthy food. He admitted that he wasn't treating his body well. His job and a new relationship consumed his schedule. He was definitely staying up too late zoning out to TV. At that appointment, I recommended lifestyle changes and ordered some labs.

At his follow-up, he had done a marvelous job adjusting lifestyle factors. He cleaned up his diet, drank water rather than soda, started walking to work, and dedicated himself to a sleep routine—whether he could fall asleep or not. He was motivated to improve his libido. But after a few months, he didn't feel much better and was still pale with dark circles under his eyes. There was an issue on his labs that I was concerned about.

A more in-depth test showed that his kidneys were in trouble. He was developing something called nephrotic syndrome—at 21! He followed adjustments to his treatment plan and we watched his labs carefully. He was very compliant and had improvements on both his tests and symptoms, but they were only mild. Normally in practice, I would've expected near complete recovery in someone so young, motivated, and otherwise healthy.

Then his mother came to see me for help with asthma attacks and fatigue. His sibling came in with fatigue, chronic sinusitis, and new food sensitivities. The whole family struggled with insomnia. There were other symptoms that led me to ask about their home environment. It turns out that they had mold in their home.

This young man chose to move out of the house in order to restore his kidney function. Within a few months, his kidneys recovered, back pain eased up, and energy improved. He no longer needed such a substantial treatment plan. At a follow-up visit, about five years after his move, he looked healthy. Libido issues were gone, and his relationship was going strong. He had no issues with fatigue unless he stayed up too late or worked too many hours—normal stuff.

Granted, initially he wasn't treating his body very well. But when someone makes positive lifestyle changes and doesn't see the benefits, more investigation is warranted. In his case, it was mold. ✸

SYMPTOMS

IMMUNE SYSTEM

- **Increased susceptibility to infection**
- **Long-lasting colds**
- **Viral infections become bacterial**
- **Chronic mono or Epstein-Barr virus**
- **Frequent Herpes outbreaks**
- **Increased susceptibility to cancer**

STORY | **CHURCH SECRETARY**

A delightful woman asked for my help with a most embarrassing problem, a lady issue. She had developed itching and burning in her lady area. She hadn't been sexually active for quite some time. She had no apparent reason for a change in this area of her body. After examination and testing, she was diagnosed with bacterial vaginosis, a flora imbalance of the vagina.

Her friends and confidants reassured her that these inconvenient changes can happen with menopause, and maybe her new job was stressing her out. She admitted that since taking the new job as church secretary, she frequently felt overwhelmed. With the pressures of learning a new job, she had gained weight but didn't necessarily eat more. Stress also caused her to have an upset stomach and digestive gas.

It turns out she was handling stress just fine. She was working in a moldy room. Mold was growing behind the paneling that lined her office.

Organizations that rely on volunteers to maintain their buildings are susceptible to mold issues. The good nature of those willing to help is hard to pass up, but not all are skilled in the trades. The problem with water is that it will exploit this inexperience and find its way into buildings.

In this woman, mold created a persistent immune depletion. What started as a yeast infection became a persistent bacterial issue as her natural flora fought to restore balance. She took antibiotics on and off for two years before the mold was discovered. It was a bacteria problem, but the underlying cause was mold.

She wasn't having respiratory symptoms because the spores were trapped behind the paneling, but the mycotoxins were getting through. The weight gain, sense of overwhelm, digestive gas and upset stomach went away when the mold was addressed. ✹

SYMPTOMS

REPRODUCTIVE SYSTEM

- Changes in menstrual cycle
- Vaginal yeast or bacterial infections
- Jock itch
- Infertility in both genders

STORY | **INFERTILITY**

This story is about the mother of the infant boy with eczema mentioned earlier. She and her husband wanted very badly to get pregnant again.

Because I didn't specialize in fertility, I referred her to colleagues. She apparently had a hard time getting pregnant with the little boy with eczema, her second child. Her first son was a four-year old with autism.

A year since finding the mold in their home, she and her husband still didn't have any luck getting pregnant. They remediated, but the mold didn't seem to want to go away. Their home required a total of three remediations. Each time they moved back, the baby boy, my patient, broke out in a rash. Mold toxins also interfered with the couple's fertility.

In this case, no one in the family felt well until they moved from the cottage with a moldy history. Even though they did the extra work of clearing mycotoxins and disposing of most of their belongings, they still couldn't get pregnant until they moved. Some people are simply too genetically sensitive to mold. There are times when the best action is to get out. ✹

LOOKS LIKE MOLD BUT ISN'T

I also work with people who have Lyme Disease. Mold follows many of the same rules as Lyme Disease.

MOLD and Lyme... imitate other conditions
can make preexisting illnesses worse
alter responses to treatments

For example, a mold-sick person may get anxiety from antianxiety medication, or insomnia from sleep medication.

If you compare symptom lists for Lyme Disease and for mold, the two lists look very similar. According to the groundbreaking work of renowned Lyme expert, Dr. Richard Horowitz, Lyme has one distinction—wandering symptoms. Lyme arthritis wanders. Lyme muscle pain wanders. Lyme nerve pain wanders.

In contrast, mold symptoms don't wander. As another distinction, mold typically affects the respiratory tract much more than Lyme. If you fill out the Crista Mold Questionnaire, and mold isn't indicated, yet you still feel lousy, I recommend the Horowitz Lyme/MSIDS Questionnaire (see *Resources* section). It just might be Lyme Disease.

CHICKEN OR EGG?

I frequently get asked the chicken or egg question about mold and Lyme. If you know you have mold sickness and also have Lyme disease (or MSIDS), which came first? One of my teachers, gifted healer, Dr. Wayne Anderson, notes that both mold and Lyme impair the immune system and increase your susceptibility to each condition. If you have mold sickness, you can more easily develop chronic or persisting Lyme disease. Conversely, if you have Lyme disease, you're more susceptible to the effects of mold.

Which came first? Dr. Wayne Anderson taught me that it doesn't matter which came first. The real question to ask is, which needs to be treated at this moment? That's the real chicken-and-egg question. The answer is a moving target. Which problem rears its ugly head at any moment will vary.

The best person to answer that question is a skilled Lyme- and mold-literate doctor. Working as your personal body translator, your doctor will read which layer needs to be addressed and pick the right treatment for this moment.

DON'T FREAK OUT

If you filled out the Crista Mold Questionnaire, and it suggests that you have mold sickness, you are probably pretty freaked out by now. You might be feeling like there's no hope, that mold wins.

NO WAY!

You are empowered with know-how. The first part of this book was all about understanding mold and learning its behaviors and weaknesses. As insurmountable as mold seems, don't get discouraged and don't give up. You have the power and the information to get better. Use the tools in this book and follow the steps. Find a mold-literate doctor to guide you. You can conquer mold and take back your health!

1.4
Diagnostics & Tests

WHAT'S IN A NAME?

What is it called when you're sick from mold? What's your official diagnosis? Well, that often depends on whether your doctor is mold-literate or not. As you see from the stories so far, your diagnosis might accurately describe your symptoms, yet the underlying cause is really mold.

Mold is only on the radar for most doctors when symptoms fit the definition of "mold allergy." This doesn't quite cut it. Allergy only accounts for "spore illness." Mold sickness is so much more than an allergy. A more expanded diagnosis is needed that encompasses mycotoxin illness, but we don't have one. In this book, I call it mold sickness, hoping by now, you understand that mold sickness is "spore" and "mycotoxin" sickness.

Leaders in the field are using descriptive terms, such as toxic mold syndrome, biotoxin illness, CIRS (Chronic Inflammatory Response Syndrome), mycotoxicosis, and on and on. But most insurance companies don't recognize these. I don't care how you name it, mold can make you sick with more than just mold spores. If that's the only tidbit you take away from this book, I've accomplished my goal.

TEST YOURSELF

If you haven't already, take time now to fill out the Crista Mold Questionnaire at the beginning of the book. Make sure to write down the date. I recommend doing this before you make any changes to your health or building. As you work through your healing process, fill it out again routinely. The questionnaire is a good way to track your progress.

HELPFUL LABORATORY TESTS

If you filled out the Crista Mold Questionnaire and are concerned that you might be sick from mold, you need more information. You can ask your doctor for the following tests. My frustration with "the system" is that many of these tests are out-of-pocket. Buyer beware.

I invite doctors who want to learn more about assessments and treatments for mold and mycotoxin illness to take my physician-level training course to understand the medical rationale in more depth.

URINE MYCOTOXINS

This easy pee test can detect mycotoxins in your urine. If the test shows that you have mycotoxins in your urine, it means either you're actively being exposed or you have misbehaving fungus in your body—or both. This simple test can help confirm that your problem is mold. It has reassured more than a few of my "canary" patients that their health problems were real.

This test is useful for tracking treatment progress as well. I've seen a connection between symptom severity and mycotoxin levels. As symptoms improve, mycotoxin levels drop, and vice-versa. As mycotoxin levels increase, symptoms worsen.

Sometimes stored mycotoxins are temporarily dumped during detox, and people have aggravations in their symptoms. This suggests a correlation between mycotoxin exposure and symptoms.

I find urine mycotoxin testing to be a very useful diagnostic tool for most mold-sick patients, but not all. A select few have such impaired detoxification systems, they can't get the toxins transported to the urine. Your doctor can try inducing them to dump, but it can definitely cause an aggravation of your symptoms.

Due to the possibility of mycotoxins in certain foods, I recommend avoiding the no-no foods and beverages listed in section *2.1 Avoidance* for three days before collecting urine for the test. This little assurance reduces the chance that if mycotoxins were found, they were from the food you ate. You should also make sure to take the first morning's collection. This test is out-of-pocket.

LABORATORY TESTS

The following laboratory tests can be used as screening tools to see if mold is affecting your body. Most are blood tests unless indicated.

PURPOSE	LABORATORY TESTS
Anemia	Complete blood count (CBC)
Allergy	Immune globulin reaction to mold (not useful for mycotoxin reactions)
Immune function	Vitamin D (25-hydroxyvitamin D) White blood cell count (WBC) Natural killer (NK) cell total count Natural killer (NK) cell function T-cell count B-cell count Transforming Growth Factor ß-1 (TGF ß-1)
Glutathione	Red blood cell glutathione
Liver health	Liver enzymes (ALT, AST, GGT)
Kidney health	Creatinine Glomerular filtration rate (GFR) Anti-diuretic hormone (ADH)
Candida overgrowth	Immune globulin reaction to Candida albicans
Genetic susceptibility	HLA-DR/DQ (DRB1, DQB1, DRB3-5)
Indicators & impacts	Organic acids urine test

One of the most specific tests that will help your doctor determine if mold is causing immune deficiency is the natural killer (NK) cell function test. This is different from the NK cell total count. NK cells are part of your immune army.

Mold expert, Dr. Joseph Brewer, first introduced me to the phenomenon that it's common for mold-sick people to have a normal NK cell total count with a low NK cell function. Your body tries to compensate for the low function by increasing total numbers. Mold is one of the few things that reduces the function or activity of natural killer cells. Not only does the NK cell function test narrow the diagnosis toward mold sickness, it's a useful test to track treatment progress.

STOOL TEST

That's right, get the scoop on your poop. A comprehensive stool assessment is a reliable method to check for fungal elements in a body. Fungal overgrowth in the gut reflects a high fungal body burden. Some labs also test to see if the fungus is sensitive to various treatments to help your doctor choose the most effective treatment.

One limitation is that this test doesn't determine what's causing the fungal overgrowth. Poor dietary choices can definitely be the sole cause. But if someone is doing everything right and still having mold symptoms that center around digestion, I'll use this test. Ask your lab how long to avoid probiotics before collecting the sample so you're getting the best information. This test is out-of-pocket.

POSTERIOR NASAL CULTURE

The utility of this test is under debate. The accuracy is questionable, and many labs don't check for certain microbes present in sinus biofilm. The test can be useful if sinusitis is the main problem and it's not responding to treatment.

No test is perfect. It's important to note that many nasal treatments make this test look normal even if it isn't. If your doctor has ordered an intranasal culture, make sure to stop all nasal washes or sprays. Long-term use of steroid sprays can also affect the accuracy. In one patient, the essential oil diffuser by her bedside was enough to make the culture negative. She stopped using it for the repeat culture, and the sinus critters were able to be found. That tells me that essential oils are good sinus antifungal tools.

SHOEMAKER

No book on mold would be complete without an homage to pioneering doctor, researcher, and mold warrior, Dr. Ritchie Shoemaker. He picked up on mold illness long before others in his field. He identified that his patients who were exposed to water-damaged buildings suffered multisystemic, multisymptomatic conditions. His astute observation propelled decades of research, innovative tests, and treatments. His tireless efforts helped to bring mold and mold toxin illness, called biotoxin illness, into the consciousness of the medical profession.

There are a host of Shoemaker lab tests that can be used to monitor mold illness. Dr. Shoemaker offers training courses on his lab tests and treatment protocols. Even though I'm not a Shoemaker-trained doctor, I will occasionally use one or two of these innovative tests to help clarify the picture or offer direction on treatment. Some of these tests are out-of-pocket.

VCS

The easiest and least invasive Shoemaker test is the Visual Contrast Sensitivity (VCS) test. Most mold sufferers flunk this functional visual acuity test. It challenges your vision and checks to see if the systems in charge of vision are up to the challenge. If not, there's a high suspicion of mold sickness. You can find this test at Dr. Shoemaker's website, Surviving Mold (see *Resources* section). The current cost is $15.

STORY | **NOT AN ALCOHOLIC**

A man in his late 50s came to see me looking for a second opinion. His doctor kept suspecting he was an alcoholic and telling him to stop drinking. Apparently there was a certain lab test that indicated alcoholism, but this man didn't drink alcohol at all. He said he'd swear on his mother's grave if he were asked to.

He originally went to the doctor with upper abdominal pain on the right side. He had episodes of nausea and would sometimes vomit. He was obese and lethargic, and he had been previously diagnosed with prediabetes.

His wife teased that he had gotten lazy after the kids moved out and he finally got his man-cave. His man-cave was one of their kid's rooms converted to an office. He would close the door and crank up the window air conditioner. He was always hot, and his wife was always cold. His office was a cool sanctuary, and he'd often fall asleep sitting at his desk.

The problematic lab test was called GGT. It's a liver enzyme that can increase with alcohol use. His other liver tests were on the rise as well, indicating an unhappy liver. He had a slowly increasing blood sugar and curiously had very, very low cholesterol.

His liver was definitely struggling. But it was not due to drinking alcohol. It was due to breathing mycotoxins. The window air conditioner was full of mold. It was decades old and had never been cleaned. He pulled it out of storage to set up his man cave. As he sat at his desk, with the door closed and air conditioner cranked, the mold and mycotoxins were polluting his air and his body. ✹

So you found out that mold is the culprit **What do you do about it?**

PART 2
THE 5 TOOLS

The Big Picture

Many of the tools can be used on your own, but I recommend finding a mold-literate doctor. Knowing which tool to use, how much, and at what stage takes a trained eye. A doctor has the advantage of a clear, mold-free mind. A doctor also has the training to catch issues that you might be blaming on mold but aren't actually from mold.

The information in this book is a beginning. You may need more rigorous or comprehensive care. Unfortunately, that's not uncommon with mold sickness because it's often diagnosed late.

In short, here are the five tools in order:

1. Avoidance
2. Fundamentals
3. Protect
4. Repair
5. Fight

PEEL THE ORANGE

I approach treatment for mold sickness in a specific order. The order isn't written in stone. It's an approach I've developed after working with many mold-sick patients. I recommend using the tools in this order to reduce suffering.

The idea of peeling an orange is the best analogy I could come up with. Like peeling an orange, you can't get to the juicy stuff until you peel the outer layers. Peel the outer orange layer first, and then the second fluffy layer to get to the sections in the middle. You work your way through each section until you've had a tasty treat. That's the same for mold.

The first two layers are necessary to be peeled completely. Others can be picked at, choosing which things will solve the problem for you personally.

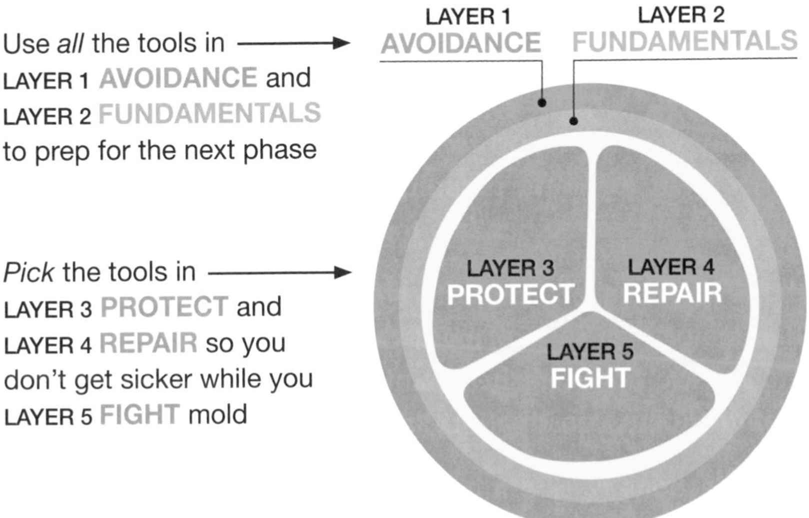

If you begin killing mold without doing any preparation, *you will get sicker*. I guarantee it. The preparation accomplished in the first few tools protects you. They're like the hazmat suits that mold remediators wear. These professionals know the hazards of going into a moldy building unprotected, so they take precautions. You need to do the same.

I've done it the wrong way. I've made patients sicker. Before I fully understood how mold impacts a body, I started patients on antifungal therapy right away, and they crashed.

Any mold symptom you're dealing with today, will get much

worse if you jump into a battle against mold without a plan or preparation.

HERX

The crash from mold is often called a Herx, or Jarisch-Herxheimer reaction. This is the concept that you can get temporarily sicker while you're working to get better. A true Herx occurs after a major mold die-off when the killed critters spill their toxic, inflammatory guts all over the place. You get sicker because your body tries to clean up the mess, but it can't keep up.

Herxing with mold tends to go right to the brain and affect your mental game. People feel hopeless, helpless, and overwhelmed. They may weep or report feeling sadder than they've ever felt in their lives, yet can't pinpoint a reason. They've described feeling out of their bodies, in a fog, and on drugs.

Other Herx reactions can affect other body systems as well: inflammatory innards of mold can cause fevers, chills, body pain, muscle aches, rashes, joint inflammation and stiffness, abdominal pain, constipation, and crampy diarrhea.

These reactions can be minimized greatly by using the tools in order.

IF IT FEELS TOO HARD, IT'S TOO HARD

I'm not a fan of "going for the Herx." I'm telling you about it to alert you to the possibility. It's not unusual to feel worse while you strive to feel better, but it's not necessary. With good preparation, you may sail through this process feeling incrementally better as you go, without a crash. Doing the preparation doesn't ensure you won't Herx. However, it definitely pushes the needle farther away from crashing.

The trend in mold and environmental medicine is to "go for the

Herx," as if a Herx is proof that we're on the right track. The thought being that the longer and more severe the Herx, the more mold we're killing. I don't buy it.

A true Herx lasts 2-3 days and then clears, sometimes requiring aid. (that's a different set of tools—covered in section *2.5 Fight*). If you have a drastic worsening of symptoms after starting some kind of treatment, and you can't move out of it after 3 days, it's too much.

Anytime it feels too hard, the plan is probably asking too much of your body. Take a pause in your push to get better. You won't lose ground. You actually might gain ground by providing necessary rest and nutrient restocking.

Rest, reflection and reassessment don't get much press in this book, but they should. Only you can know when to push pause. Trust yourself.

DON'T GO HOG WILD

If you've been inspired to make a bunch of changes and take back your health, awesome. Do me a favor, though. Don't stop any medications.

I saw this in practice. Enthused about finding the answer to her mysterious suffering, a patient assumes the first step is to stop all her medications cold turkey and go all natural. The results were catastrophic.

Please, please, please resist the temptation to stop your medications! This is all the more important if you're taking steroid or immune-suppressive medication. You may eventually be able to trim the dose or stop a medication as a result of treating the cause. If the cause is mold, many suppressive medications are no longer necessary after you've been treated. But you have to crowd out the need for the medication with resounding health and vitality. Rely on your doctor to decide when that step can be taken.

HEALING DOESN'T WORK IN A STRAIGHT LINE

I can't tell you how many times I've said this to my patients. We want healing to be an orderly process, but it just isn't. When I try to describe what healing really looks like, I end up describing a Celtic knot and using all kinds of hand gestures. One day I gave up, and scratched something down on paper.

Are you ready? Today's your lucky day! I dug out a hand-drawn image of how healing really works that I drew for a patient; it's not elegant but gets the point across.

On the left is what we want healing to look like: steady, forward, upward progress and continuous improvement. On the right is what healing really looks like: overall forward progress and improvement, but with lots of circling back to clear old gunk.

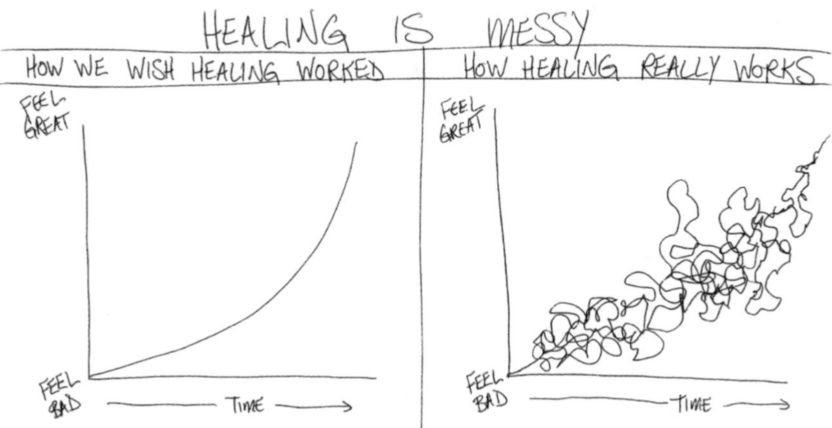

Healing from chronic disease works differently than healing from acute disease. When you get a cold, the best remedy is to rest and recoup: stay in bed, sleep, hydrate, eat very little, and your body will steadily display fewer and fewer uncomfortable symptoms. When you're coming back from a chronic illness like mold sickness, the best remedy is to stand up and fight: get out of bed, move your body, seek clean environments, eat specific foods, and work the plan, and your body will heal in fits and spurts.

The goal is to have fewer bad moments and more good moments so that the bad moments get "less bad" while the good moments get "more good." If this is happening, keep working your plan. It's working. Don't overthink it.

HEALING IS MESSY

A human's body language can be very confusing. You may be 100% on your healing path, but your most annoying symptom doesn't seem to be improving. Or suddenly you develop a really disruptive symptom, which might leave you feeling like you're being punished for doing the right thing.

The body has an internal order of operations. It prioritizes the most critical body systems first, then goes for the next vital, and so on.

Quiz time!

Which is more vital to basic human survival if injured: the brain or the skin?

If you answered the brain, you're thinking like a human body. I use these two examples purposefully.

It's quite common to see a skin rash develop in someone who's been sick from mold for a long time with brain-related symptoms. Parkinson's-like tremors get incrementally better, just as a new rash appears. The body pushes the mycotoxins from the central nervous system out to the outer-most layers of the body—the skin—which causes a rash. That's your body thanking you! Odd, huh?

If you're doing it right, your body will use its newfound fuel to push the mold and mycotoxins from the deep systems to the surface ones, from the vital organs to those that help clean things up, and from the most damaging to the least damaging.

If your eyes have cleared up (vision is important for survival), but you develop foot fungus (irritating but not affecting basic survival), then you're on the right path.

If your balance has improved (brain function) but the post-nasal drip you used to have is back (irritation), then things are moving in the right direction.

As you peel back the layers of the orange, you often clear an old symptom. Quite often, the symptom is cleared by activating it, which isn't necessarily bad news. Healing is messy and disorderly. Look at basic body functions to judge how you're doing—energy, sleep, digestion, and mood. If your basic bodily functions are improving, stick to the plan.

LOW-HANGING FRUIT

If you're sick from mold, you're likely overwhelmed. The prospect of reading this book was probably more than you could handle, let alone taking any action. I get it. Go for the low-hanging fruit.

Get out of the environment. That alone can help your energy and clarity. Then take the next step—make a plan.

> Wars Are Fought **One Battle At a Time**

Be gentle with yourself. Be realistic. There's no perfect way to do this. Do one achievable thing at a time, and then wait. Take it slow. Any movement toward health is helpful. Just don't give up. **You CAN get better!**

2.1 Avoidance

This entire layer of the orange, every suggestion in this section, is necessary. The recommendations in this layer are basic requirements. They set the foundation for the rest of the tools to work best.

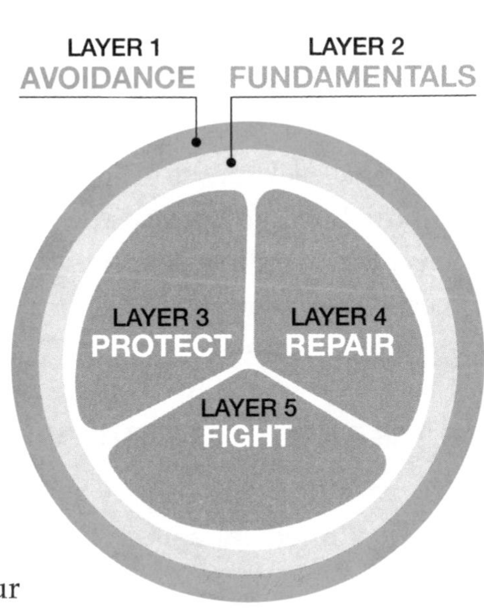

Every aspect of AVOIDANCE is required to regain your health from mold. Those that put on blinders and "avoid avoidance" have delays, set-backs, and reduced response to treatment. Some simply don't get better.

Before you begin any changes, fill out the Crista Mold Questionnaire and note the date. This is your baseline. After you've peeled this layer of the orange, take it again. You'll be surprised how much can improve with the AVOIDANCE tool.

AVOIDANCE

According to my environmental medicine instructor and guru of all things detox, Dr. Walter Crinnion, these are the absolute first 3 rules of toxic indoor exposures:

1 AVOIDANCE

2 AVOIDANCE

3 AVOIDANCE

Get the point?

That's right, avoiding exposure to mold is so important, it takes up the first three steps.

AVOIDANCE 1 **GET OUT!**

AVOIDANCE 2 **TAKE NOTHING WITH YOU**

AVOIDANCE 3 **PREVENT EXPOSURES**

1 GET OUT!

Leave the sick environment with an open-ended duration. Construction has a way of taking longer than expected. To prevent frustration, expect it to take longer than quoted. Check your insurance policy to see if it covers your temporary relocation, many do.

2 TAKE NOTHING WITH YOU

Take as little with you as possible, not even the favorites—favorite stuffed animals, favorite pillows, etc. Your "things" can take on mold spores and mold toxins.

③ PREVENT EXPOSURES

Remediate your environment, your diet, and your habits. Mold-sick people tend to be attracted to moldy spaces, moldy foods, and mold-supportive hobbies. That's because if you stop feeding the mold in your body, it starts to die, spill its guts, and make you sick. So you feed it. But don't.

Okay, you may be wondering, how are you supposed to avoid mold if it's living in your sinuses? Remember that part in the beginning, "if you have mold sickness, you take the problem with you wherever you go—in your sinuses?" You don't "avoid" sinus mold. You kill it. But not until you have your prep done.

DON'T COOK YOUR OWN FROG

What did I do when I found out we had mold in our home? I'm a trained mold doctor, so of course I got my family out of dodge…right?

Nope. I stayed! And we got sick.

Can you believe that? Even after I found out it was mold, we stayed in the environment. We kept living there because I underestimated the scope of our problem. By doing that, we got sick. Our frogs slowly got cooked!

Of all the environmentally ill patients I've worked with, mold-sick patients are the most resistant to the idea that mold is the problem. They're also the most stubborn about leaving their moldy environments. I'm a classic case-in-point. I've done a lot of soul-searching about that. Because I underestimated my mold issue, I didn't get myself and my family out of the house. How did I join the ranks of my mold-sick patients and not leave my sick home?

I alluded to it earlier. When you leave the sick environment, the mold in your sinuses and digestive tract loses its community. It begins to die. And like I talked about earlier, mold doesn't go down without a fight. As mold dies, mycotoxins are spilled into your body at a higher rate. As more mycotoxins are spilled, you feel worse. They're usually not obvious symptoms but more like brain fog, fatigue, distractibility, irritability, or sweet cravings.

That's why mold-sick people seem unable to leave the environment, and why they tend toward attracting more mold. It's mold's Jedi mind trick to turn you into food. Avoidance of mold-promoting environments, foods, drinks, and habits is the first step toward conquering mold.

In a nutshell, here are the categories of AVOIDANCE...

1 Habitat
2 Air Quality
3 Foods To Avoid
4 Beverages To Avoid
5 Supplement & Medication Cautions
6 Hobbies & Habits

1 HABITAT

Distrust must. If a place smells musty, run away. Even if it doesn't smell funny, if a location causes ANY mold symptom to reoccur, get out. Remember that mold makes you sick with both spores and gases, and the dangerous, most toxic gases don't have a scent. But if you smell a musty, mildewy smell, you know for sure there's mold.

Getting out of the sick environment is important, but fixing that space is key. This is called remediation. Remediation means that the moisture source is corrected and sick materials are removed. I talk more about remediation in *Part 3—Buildings*.

2 AIR QUALITY

Seek clean air. Indoor air quality is commonly worse than outdoor air quality. For this reason, I'm a big fan of appropriate air filtration. All air filters are not created equal, however. I've listed my favorites in the Resources section. When it comes to mold recovery, you need an air filter that not only traps spores, but also cleans mycotoxins.

Remember the lung picture in section *1.1—Hidden Agenda*? It shows that mycotoxins are teeny tiny and can absorb through the lungs and into the body. You want a room air filter that can filter down to the mycotoxin level, as small as 0.1 microns.

Avoid any air filter that spits out ozone. Ozone is harmful to respiratory passages. However, sanitizing air filters that pump out ionized oxygen are okay.

For the chemistry-curious, the oxygen we breathe is made up of two oxygen molecules happily bound together. Ozone is made up of three oxygen molecules—a real three's-a-crowd problem. The extra oxygen molecule desires to find its own coupling. If it finds a compatibility, it will push others out of the way, which is destructive to the balance of other chemical bonds. This "oxidation" causes tissue destruction. If inhaled, it can harm lung tissue.

Ionized oxygen is different. Ionized oxygen makes the fresh scent of waterfalls, oceanfronts, and line-dried sheets. Ionized oxygen is normal oxygen (two molecules) with a little added energy. Ionized (or energized) oxygen is safe for the lungs and is very generous. Ionized oxygen transfers its extra energy to our bodies and easily absorbs into the deeper tissues—where mycotoxins can go. If you can't live near the ocean or some other natural creator of ionized oxygen, a sanitizing air filter is a good substitute.

A good air filter is NOT a replacement for remediation. A square inch of mold contains nearly 1 million spores. One million spores kick out 500 million fragments. Mycotoxins are then released from 501 million mycotoxin-forming spores and parts. That amounts to many balloons-full of toxic gas released into your indoor air on a daily basis.

> Air Filtration **Is Not a Replacement** For Remediation

There's no amount of air filtration, open windows, or fans that can keep up with this degree of mycotoxins. That's more toxic gas bombs than any air filter can take care of. You have to do the remediation. The air filtration is simply a tool to protect you from any possible cross-contamination from remediation.

STORY | **C-PAP DEMENTIA**

I was visited by concerned adult children of a long-time patient in her late 70s. Their mom was beginning to show signs of dementia. A fully independent go-getter, she apparently had started to forget things, like closing the garage door overnight, which made her kids worry about safety.

She seemed more and more confused, and was having balance issues. Her 76-year-old husband was fine, other than griping about having to use a C-PAP machine at bedtime for his sleep apnea. She too used a C-PAP for insomnia due to restless leg syndrome.

After ruling out other potential causes and doing a home visit, my concern grew about mold. They lived in a historic home, and they admitted to being bad about dusting. We added a good quality air filter in the bedroom. His insomnia improved. Hers worsened.

She described having high anxiety at night. She worried and fretted, and trivial things seemed insurmountable. She'd also lose track of where she was. She reported sleeping like a baby in another area of house for her daily nap—a location too far from her C-PAP to use it. I began to suspect her C-PAP machine. On testing, the mold inspector found high amounts of Aspergillus in her C-PAP machine. There was nothing detected in her husband's machine.

When asked about maintenance, she admitted she was very good at maintaining her husband's but frequently skipped cleaning her own because she only had restless legs, not trouble breathing like her husband. When tubing was replaced and the machine cleaned appropriately, dementia symptoms slowly disappeared. ✹

3 FOODS TO AVOID

If you've held it together until now, good for you. Now I'm going to mess with your sacred cows—your favorite foods and beverages.

Take comfort, these only need to be avoided during mold treatment. After you're out of the sick environment and have cleared the effects of toxic mold from your body, you'll likely be able to reintroduce them. See the *Reintroduction* section in *2.5—Fight*.

AVOID

FOODS FIRST TIER

- Sweets of any kind
- Dried fruits
- Leavened bread
- Yeast
- Simple carbohydrates
- Baked goodies
- Mushrooms
- Corn
- Potatoes
- Pickles & pickled foods
- Vinegar
- Soy sauce
- Cantaloupe
- Grapes
- Aged cheeses
- Moldy cheeses
- Peanuts
- Peanut butter

Avoiding foods in the first tier works for most people, those that get out of the sick environment. Their symptoms reduce and they get a leg up on mold. But some people need more.

They feel much better on a more restrictive diet. The only way to know for sure is trial and error.

AVOID

FOODS SECOND TIER

- **All fruit**
- **Starchy vegetables**
- **All grains**
- **Fermented foods**
- **Shelled nuts**
- **Condiments made with vinegar or sugar**
- **Sour cream or other soured milk products**

If you feel better avoiding both the first and second tier, you may also have candida overgrowth in your intestines. Candida is a yeast that's normally found in the digestive tract. Like colonization of the sinuses, peacefully coexisting yeast starts to behave badly after exposure to a water-damaged building.

Yeasts and molds are in the fungus family. I think of candida overgrowth as fungal overload of the gut. The yeast makes toxins that are similar to the mold toxins from a water-damaged building. Typically, foods that feed yeast also feed mold colonies.

The Internet has a plethora of anti-candida diets. You may notice that they look similar to my list but not the same. Some foods are missing from my list. I've purposefully only included foods on my no-no list that are mold and yeast specific. In other words, they either contain molds and mycotoxins, or they promote fungal overgrowth. Other lists expand to include general healthy diet recommendations. While I applaud the comprehensiveness, mold-sick people are already overwhelmed. I'm going to stick to mold.

4 BEVERAGES TO AVOID

This section is going to crush a lot of you. Apologies in advance. Remember, it's likely temporary.

AVOID

BEVERAGES

ANY sweetened beverage
Fruit juice
Oolong and black tea (partially fermented)
Moldy coffee (check that your company has independent testing)
Alcoholic beverages
Fermented beverages, such as cider, kombucha

I'm frequently asked to explain my rationale for putting kombucha on the AVOIDANCE list. It's supposed to promote health by balancing gut bacteria, so it seems perfect on paper. Unfortunately, it also feeds mold. Daily kombucha has been the barrier to improvement for a number of patients. I've seen one glass of kombucha cause bloating, cramping, fatigue, and crippling brain fog in a mold-sick person.

A little tip on food and beverage avoidance—plan ahead for social events. Bring alternatives, alert hosts, and come up with simple one-liners to use when people want to pressure you into eating or drinking things that could make you sick. Say something simple like, "no thanks," or "that doesn't make me feel good," or "sorry, I'm allergic," or "some crazy lady who wrote a mold book told me not to eat that." Keep it simple and move on. I'm sorry to be blunt and honest, but no one wants to hear the whole saga in a social setting, yet you need to protect yourself. Come up with something that works for you in advance, use it when needed, and move on.

5 SUPPLEMENT & MEDICATION CAUTIONS

Certain supplements have the potential to make a mold-sick person feel worse.

SUPPLEMENTS to avoid... are actual fungus
are grown on mold
contain mycotoxins

An innovative technique being used in the supplement industry uses mold, usually Aspergillus, to extract active constituents out of plant material. In theory, it makes the nutrient bio-activated and more useful to the body. The problem is that mold-sick people can't tolerate anything that's been within 10 feet of mold, let alone grown on it.

If you have a supplement that's been extracted, processed, or activated using fungus, you likely won't be able to tolerate it. Many B-vitamins fall into this category. If you aren't mold sensitive, it's not a problem. After you're out of the environment and treated for mold sickness, it's not a problem. But while you're having symptoms, I recommend avoiding supplements that have been processed or fermented with Aspergillus, fungus, yeast or mold.

Medicinal mushrooms in theory would be perfect for mold sickness to repair the immune depletion that mold creates. Sadly, when you are actively mold-sick, they can make you sicker by tipping the scale toward fungal overgrowth. Once out of the sick environment and treated, medicinal mushrooms are a fantastic tool to rebalance the immune system.

The same goes for Saccharomyces boulardii. This yeast is added to probiotic blends to combat candida overgrowth. It's a safe yeast that shoves candida out of the gut yet can't colonize in it. You poop it out once its job is done. This is another one that in theory is perfect, but in practice, has caused my mold-sick patients to flare. Many of my colleagues will disagree. I speak from my own experience.

AVOID

SUPPLEMENTS FUNGAL OVERLOAD

Saccharomyces boulardii

Nutritional yeast

Medicinal mushrooms

AVOID

SUPPLEMENTS GROWN WITH YEAST/MOLD

Aspergillus-activated brands

Some B-vitamin brands

AVOID

SUPPLEMENTS MAY CONTAIN MYCOTOXIN

Red yeast rice

(use only companies that conduct independent testing)

Bee propolis

Make sure you're not taking any supplements that are contaminated with mycotoxins. Most reputable supplement companies regularly test and control for mycotoxin contamination.

CAUTION

MEDICATIONS TWO CATEGORIES

Antibiotics: many classes of antibiotics are mycotoxins. They're based on the antibacterial effect of mold mycotoxins. Use these types of antibiotics only if necessary. Try others first if an antibiotic is needed.

Strong antifungal herbs and medications: take caution using these without prepping your body first.

6 HOBBIES & HABITS

Mold-sick people tend to be attracted to activities and spaces that promote mold survival—think historic restoration, brewmaster, breadmaker, cheese connoisseur, rare book collector, thrift shop worker, hoarder, and so forth. I believe this is mold's trick to keep itself alive. I'm not saying every brewmaster is sick with mold. I'm saying if you ARE sick from mold, pay attention to how you feel as you move through your life.

Take a look at your habit, or your hobby. Is it a passion? Or are you beholden to it?

TRUST YOURSELF

If you're having reactions in certain spaces, listen to your body. If you feel cruddy after eating certain food, listen to your body. You rarely go wrong listening to your body.

Your reactions are sure to be inconveniences to you and those around you. It will be tempting to ignore these messages, and it will be tempting to medicate them if you can't ignore them. People around you will be happy to have you ignore those messages. Your reactions are probably forcing change in others' lives. The "canaries in the coal mine" people, the first to react, often get disbelieved or blown-off by others as a reaction to resist change. We hate change. Change is uncomfortable, but so is getting sick.

When our first remediation was complete in my house, I felt a sense of accomplishment. I had conquered the problem before we got really sick. As I got better and stronger, I was able to discern how I felt in specific areas of my house. Unfortunately, my kitchen was still a problem area. I felt foggy and exhausted, and my lungs would begin to burn.

Trusting my body, I scheduled a full, messy, inconvenient

demolition of the tile floor and any affected cabinets. I asked for samples of everything, including the cement board. I was told it was unnecessary, that cement board under tile didn't grow mold. But I was having reactions to it. After removing it, the remediators graciously went along with my request and provided a chunk to send in for testing. Sure thing, it came back infected with two different kinds of mold. The remediators were stunned. They were taught differently. They were interested in this new knowledge, and the fact that my "canary" sensitivity was validated by science. I'm extremely grateful for my training and to have learned to trust my body.

Trust yourself. If something's making you feel bad, avoid it.

2.2

Fundamentals

Just like the AVOIDANCE layer, all parts of the FUNDAMENTALS layer are recommended. This layer is the starting place for almost any health concern but is especially helpful to mold-sick people. Mold messes up the basic systems and rhythms of the body in a fundamental way. This section helps regulate them again. Once adopted, the FUNDAMENTALS become a lifestyle and second nature, rather than a chore. Make it a goal to add one section per week.

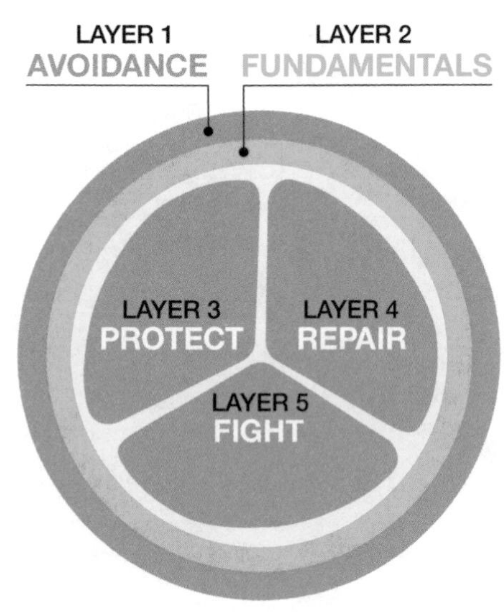

Aspects of the FUNDAMENTALS... 1 Circadian Rhythm
2 Emunctories
3 Health "Hokey Pokey"

1 CIRCADIAN RHYTHM

Circadian rhythm essentially means daily body rhythm, like an inner clock. It dictates many of our automatic body systems; processes that happen in the background without our conscious direction. We don't have to think about them or direct them, yet they happen anyway. Examples are digesting food, making tears to hydrate our eyes, pumping blood through the heart, healing a cut, getting sleepy, and so on. Believe it or not, these types of body activities are driven by nature's cycles and the seasons.

Unfortunately, the farther we've gotten from nature, the more confused those systems have become. A prime example is sleep. Normally, when the sun goes down and light fades, we get sleepy. But artificial lighting overrides this natural cycle and can cause sleep problems. Mold makes the problem even worse by altering inner circadian rhythms.

The study of these rhythms, known as chronology, shows that each system works best if allowed to fully function at its best time of day or night. It's the difference between pushing a boulder up or down a hill. Doesn't downhill sound easier?

Dr. Dietrich Klinghardt successfully treats "untreatable" chronic diseases. He's developed an effective testing and treatment approach called Autonomic Response Testing (ART). He teaches that good health is dependent first and foremost on a well-functioning autonomic nervous system. Otherwise, any other additions to the treatment plan will be stunted.

In my experience, the closer my patients adhered to nature's cycles, the faster they got better.

Here are my BASIC RECOMMENDATIONS...

- Wake within the same hour every day.
- Go to sleep within the same hour every day.
- Adjust sleep and wake times for seasonal variation in sunlight and darkness. As much as possible, let nature's light dictate when you wake and sleep.
- Eat meals at nearly the same times every day. Aim to eat most of your food earlier in the day versus later.
- Exercise within the same hour every day—the earlier in the day the better.
- Go to bed "not full," but with a little room left in your tummy.
- Give yourself time every morning to be on the toilet for regular bowel evacuation. 10 minutes minimum. Schedule it.

BACK TO NATURE, back to health.

2 EMUNCTORIES

This funny word describes a very important overall concept for health. Emunctories are body systems that excrete waste. Without them, we'd be floating in our own waste—yuck! Emunctories are involved in our embarrassing bodily functions: peeing, pooping, sweating, exhaling, making mucous, ejaculating, and menstruating. Yep, things we don't really like to talk openly about. But, they're necessary for a clean, healthy, waste-free body.

> **Well-Functioning Emunctories** Are Critical For Mold Healing

Mold mycotoxins soak into the body and end up in the lymph system. The lymph system is like our sewer system. Cells dump their waste into the lymph, or sewer lines. The sewer lines are pumped clean when we move our muscles and when we sweat. The waste is collected in lymph nodes. The collected bodily waste is delivered to specific organs to be eliminated. These organs package the waste to be carried out in feces, much like we bag our garbage and put it out for the garbage trucks to take away.

Usually this system works well to clean our bodies of waste. But mold toxins overwhelm the sewer lines, taxing our elimination systems. It simply makes too many toxins. All those toxins need somewhere to go, or they backup just like a sewer into your cells. Your body needs to get them out or it becomes poisoned.

To heal from mold, you need the ins and outs of the emunctories to function.

3 HEALTH "HOKEY POKEY"

Let's cover all the basic ins and outs:

- A Air in
- B Air out
- C Air moved all about
- D Water in
- E Water out
- F Water moved all about
- G Food in
- H Food out
- I Food moved all about

You're going to feel like you're doing the health "Hokey Pokey." Hey, I'm fine with that as long as you turn your health around. That's what this whole book is all about!

Ⓐ AIR IN

To defeat mold, you absolutely must nourish this core body need. Here's my general reasoning:

Human bodies can... go without food **30** days
go without water **3** days
go without oxygen **3** minutes

What do you think is the most important priority to heal from mold? **Oxygen!**

And then? **Water!**

You got the idea.

Where do we get oxygen? **Air!**

My argument is that we shouldn't be pondering which food to eat or supplement to take if we don't have oxygen and water squarely on board.

This section is titled *Air In*. Simply put, that means…breathe.

I was amazed in practice how often I had to remind people to breathe. Are you breathing now? Like really breathing? Slow and deep and relaxed? Take a moment to pay attention. Likely not. In fact, scientific statistics say that under-breathing is at epidemic proportions. Generally, most people in the developed world are terrible breathers, and mold-sick people are the worst.

If you've been exposed to a water-damaged building, your smart body has made an adaptation you may not be aware of. Your lungs have adapted your breathing rate and depth to limit how much air you take in, to limit how much mold toxin you inhale. Your body protects you from further exposure by slowing down your breathing rate and making it more shallow. Mold-sick people inhale only to top off the tank. And if you have asthma, you also don't exhale well.

So breathe. It doesn't cost a thing. There are some great apps designed to remind you. Use them.

Ⓑ AIR OUT

To take a deep breath in, you must first make room. You need to exhale. I find that lots of people hold their breath. Yoga is my go-to for learning how to breathe out. Many yoga breathing techniques involve more time breathing out than in. This has to do with how we're wired. A long, slow purposeful exhale enhances relaxation and renewal, and resets many of our circadian rhythms.

The other aspect of *Air Out* is getting air from the *outside*. I mentioned that indoor air quality is worse than outdoor air quality in most areas of the country. Not only is outside air cleaner, it's super-charged. Outside air is ionized, meaning it's more generous with its oxygen than stale indoor air. Get time outdoors every day.

Outside also exposes you to the sun. The sun provides two mold-fighting aspects, UV light and vitamin D. UV light from the sun is mold's kryptonite. Toxic indoor molds can't survive in UV light from the sun. They wither away in the sunlight like vampires. Sunshine is a mold-fighting resource and it's free.

Sunlight also boosts our vitamin D. Vitamin D is important for our immune system, our army against mold. Vitamin D can boost the immune system's ability to recognize that mold is the problem. This is so important I'll say it again, get outside every, every, every day. Once more, every day.

Forest Bathing: The Japanese have pioneered research on the importance of getting outside. They've coined the term "forest bathing", or in Japanese, "shin rin yoku". They found that a certain branch of our immune army is boosted when we spend time outside with trees. Tree huggers are on to something!

When we spend a half hour or more outdoors appreciating trees, our immune system gets jacked up to more than double its normal size. And not only does the total number of immune fighters increase, they become better at fighting. Hanging out with trees makes our immune system more stealth.

The branch of our immune army stimulated by trees are called natural killer (NK) cells. NK cells specialize in certain immune system tasks, such as fighting cancer and—you guessed it—killing mold. Mold must know this, because it not only reduces our total NK cell count but also reduces the function of each one. In other words, it makes the soldiers forget their training.

To check to see if this branch of your immune system has been affected by mold, you can ask your doctor to run two labs: NK cell total count and NK cell function. (Discussed in section *1.5 Diagnostics & Tests*) If either is low, getting outside with trees every day is vital for you to get better.

Ⓒ AIR MOVED

I suspect that the "Hokey Pokey" says to "move it all about" in order to tire out children with too much energy. In the case of the health "Hokey Pokey" for mold, movement is necessary to *create* energy, not use it up.

Movement is important for two reasons: moving oxygen in, and moving waste out. It's one thing to breathe, but you have to move that good air around to get any use out of it. Have you ever tried to start a campfire that just won't light? Do you know how to get it to burn better? You fan the flames.

Think of movement as fanning the flames of your metabolism. Metabolism is energy. It's body fire. And it's oxygen dependent. This energy, or fire, burns up mold toxins—but not completely.

Then you have to get the charred toxins out of the body through movement. Movement delivers mold toxins to the emunctories to be excreted.

Did you notice I say "movement" and not "exercise"? I'm doing this on purpose. Exercise is intimidating. Exercise always seems to require some amount of expertise, a teacher, a membership, certain outfits, ugh . . . I'm exhausted just thinking about it.

Whereas "movement" means just that—movement. It doesn't matter how, just move. Movement can be golfing, gardening, sweeping, mowing, shoveling, sanding, cleaning, dancing, boxing, fencing, walking, bouncing on a mini-trampoline, taking the stairs, biking, rowing, going uphill, and anything else that makes you move and maybe makes you sweat. Pump the lymphatic sewers of your body clean.

If you're too sick for anything vigorous, take hot baths, wrap up in blankets, go to the steam room, or get a massage. Then rinse with a cool shower. A cool shower after warming up your body moves your blood around. Moving your blood around is almost as powerful as moving your body around. So breathe good air, and move it around.

D WATER IN

Here's a line I want you to memorize—drilled into me by environmental medicine specialists, Dr. Walter Crinnion and Dr. Lyn Patrick: **The solution to pollution is dilution.**

How do you dilute a gunky body? Flood it with clean water. Wash it on the inside. Rinse it clean and dilute the pollutants.

Hydrate, hydrate, hydrate. If you don't dilute mold toxins, they stick around and make you sick.

I recommend spring water—not reverse osmosis water, not

alkaline water, not distilled water, not purified water—only spring water. Spring water contains naturally occurring elements that help hold water in your tissues. Spring water takes the long path through the body, whereas those other types of water take the shortcut, especially for moldies.

If you have mold exposure, you pee water out almost as fast as you drink it. Mold interferes with the way the body recycles water in the kidneys. You need spring water to counter this effect.

Drink half your body weight in ounces of spring water every day. A half-gallon is 64 ounces. You need to drink a half-gallon each day if you weigh 128 pounds. You need to drink more if you weigh more.

My weight in pounds = ______
My weight cut in half = ______ = Ounces of **water** **needed** daily

E WATER OUT

Water out means exactly what you think it means—go pee-pee. After exposure to a water-damaged building, you spill mycotoxins through the urine. If you hold it, you expose your bladder wall to these toxins. Bladders don't like this. They get injured and they get irritable. If you held it, even though the toxin has moved on, the damage has been done. Your injured bladder will now tell you again and again that you have to pee, even if you don't, giving you a very overactive bladder.

Mold also reduces your kidneys' ability to retain water in the body. We make something called anti-diuretic hormone that tells the kidneys to keep some water in your blood system to maintain blood pressure. After mold exposure, the kidneys get deaf to this hormone. The result is frequent urination and increased thirst. It's very common to see urinary frequency and irritable bladder symptoms with mold sickness. Try not to fight the urge to go. It will settle down with treatment.

F WATER MOVED

A helpful way to move water is sweat. Even though it's socially inconvenient, sweating is a very important part of conquering mold. Remember, the easiest way mycotoxins enter the body is through the skin. A regular flood of sweat rids your skin of anything on the surface that wants to enter.

There's also the glorious sauna. Sauna therapy can release stored mycotoxins.

BUT saunas shouldn't be used this early in the process.

I don't recommend using sauna therapy until you have all of the FUNDAMENTALS in place, some amount of protection (see the PROTECT section), and have reduced symptoms. Only then is it okay to add another straw to the camel's back.

Reminder—hydrate!

G FOOD IN

With all that talk in the last section about what *not* to eat, I should probably suggest what *to* eat. There are lots of foods that can protect you from mold and mycotoxins. Some foods protect tissues, and some fight mold. I've given you the lists below, but here are the general rules of thumb for what to eat:

Rainbow of color
Veggies rule
Feed your guts
Say yes to good fats
Eat stinky foods

Rainbow of Color: The colorful pigments in vegetables and fruits are called bioflavonoids. Colorful bioflavonoids protect from the damaging effects of mycotoxins all over the body. Aim to eat the entire rainbow of colors in vegetables and fruits every day.

Veggies Rule: I would rather you eat way more vegetables than fruit. Fruits contain more sugars than vegetables. Mold-sick people may get fungal overgrowth problems after eating too much fruit, whereas vegetables have the colorful bioflavonoids and less sugar. On the other hand, if you need a little something sweet and are choosing between straight-up candy or fruit, go with the fruit.

Veggies also have fiber. Fiber is necessary to bind up mycotoxins, and it also maintains healthy flora in the gut.

Feed Your Guts: Certain parts of our guts need special dietary attention with mold sickness: the liver, the kidneys, and the intestines. Love your liver with specific liver-loving food, such as beets, garlic, onions, eggs, and beef liver (organic only!). Most liver-loving foods also love the kidneys. For the intestines, choose foods that feed the lining of the digestive system, such as cabbage, yogurt, and butter.

Say Yes To Good Fats: Good fats feed the bone marrow and immune system, the brain and nervous system, the organs, and glands. Good fats refer to essential fatty acids (EFAs). You may have heard of a type of these called omega-3s. There are others, named DHA, EPA, and CoQ10, which I talk about in the next chapters. EFAs can be found in foods like olive oil, avocado, fresh seeds and nuts, and fish.

Eat Stinky Foods: Stinky foods such as garlic, onions, and spices have antifungal properties. They kill yeasts and molds. My brilliant botanical medicine instructor, Dr. Jillian Stansbury, taught us to "use spices with wild abandon." I've listed spices that help fight mold and mycotoxins. One spice blend deserves special mention, which is curry. Curry is usually based around an herb called turmeric. Turmeric is a particularly powerful protector of the brain, liver, and kidneys against mycotoxins.

EAT!

PROTECTIVE FOODS

Colorful vegetables (eat more veggies than fruit)

- **Beets, artichoke, asparagus, radishes** (helps the liver)
- **Broccoli, Brussel sprouts** (detox via sulfurophanes)
- **Tomatoes** (lycopene neutralizes mycotoxins)
- **Cabbage** (helps your intestines)
- **Celery, cucumber** (helps kidneys with water balance)
- **Bitter greens such as arugula, broccoli rabe, endive, watercress, kale, dandelion greens** (detox mycotoxins)

Colorful fruits (eat more veggies than fruit)

Beef liver (use organic only)

Essential fats:

- **Avocado**
- **Olives**
- **Olive oil**
- **Fresh seeds and nuts** (refrigerate these to preserve)
- **Eggs**
- **Fish**

Yogurt (rebalance flora)

Butter (heal intestinal lining)

Healing spices:

- **Curry** (turmeric)
- **Parsley**

EAT!

MOLD FIGHTING FOODS

Garlic
Onions
Scallions
Chives
Leeks

EAT!

MOLD FIGHTING SPICES

Clove
Cumin
Rosemary
Sage
Thyme
Oregano
Basil
Bay leaf

EAT!

BITTER DRINKS & TREATS

Green tea (protective polyphenols)
Coffee
Bitter chocolate (unsweetened)

Green tea is high in something called polyphenols, which is a bioflavonoid in the same family as colorful vegetables. Polyphenols offer specific protection from the damaging effects of mold and mycotoxins.

Ⓗ FOOD OUT

What goes in must come out...**ideally 12-18 hours later**. Too soon, and you might not get all the nutrients from your food.

Too late, and you could be basking in mycotoxins. Extended mycotoxin exposure can damage the lining of your intestines. And, the longer mycotoxins sit around, the greater the chance that they'll reabsorb into circulation.

If you've ever had an appointment with a naturopathic doctor, I'm betting you've had long discussions about poop; how often, what color, what form, did it sink or float, and on and on. When it comes to your scat, specifics matter. We can tell a lot about your overall health by what comes out of your hind end.

Patients often reported to me that they had "normal" bowel movements. Yet they only went every other day. That's too slow. Toxins are surely reabsorbing at that pace. What you call "normal" may not actually be healthy.

When it comes to mold, we want people pooping 2 to 3 times every day. Try to achieve this through hydration, exercise, and fiber, rather than being "coffee regular." If that doesn't work, then add the bitters (see the *Bile Movers* subsection in the PROTECT section).

Poop is the goal!

❶ FOOD MOVED

Mold is tough on the gut. From the mouth down, it can thin the lining of our digestion, cause irritation, tire out the immune surveillance, and take over the population of our flora. Our gut flora, called our microbiome, determines our health status.

With mold sickness, rather than host beneficial bacteria to boost health, our microbiome begins to serve as a reservoir for bad-guy colonization and "dis-ease." This stubborn biofilm layer plays out like Mad Max—every microbe for itself, each competing for the top.

Probiotics can be used to reestablish a healthy microbiome. I call probiotics "enforced gentrification," supplementing only a select group of characters to inhabit your gut. Sometimes you need this extra infusion of good fellas when you're dealing with a colony similar to Mad Max. Probiotics help with regularity by restoring the right characters. Things move along as they should, and the bad guys are pooped out to "sleep with the fishes."

However, occasionally adding more good fellas just adds to the mess. If things aren't moving along as they should, your body may have forgotten how. Peristalsis (the movement of food through the intestines) becomes paralysis. This is a condition called Small Intestinal Bowel Overgrowth (SIBO), which is commonly seen with mold-sick people.

SIBO can be due to many factors. I want you to know about it because of how common it is with moldies. If probiotics cause bloating, gas, and discomfort, you may have SIBO. If so, you need special probiotics and treatment. My go-to resource people for this are Drs. Allison Siebecker and Steven Sandberg-Lewis. Watch for Dr. Siebecker's upcoming book, *The SIBO Book*, and check out her courses in the *Resources* section.

GENETICALLY WIRED TO BE A CANARY

Mold sickness is a "canary illness". Canary illnesses are caused by environmental insults that affect everyone, but some people worse than others, even at small doses. The people most affected are like canaries in the coal mine, put there to warn others about the toxic dangers. Canary people are wired differently from other people. It's genetics. Their genetics make them really bad at getting rid of the toxin, so it builds up and creates a reaction.

If you find yourself reacting to mold earlier or more severely than others, you might be genetically wired to be a mold canary.

There are things you probably need to do that go beyond the scope of this book. My go-to resource for this information is a book called *Dirty Genes* by Dr. Benjamin Lynch. Check out the *Resources* section for more information.

2.3

Protect

Remember the picture of the orange? It shows that you need to peel the outer two layers completely to access the inner sections. PROTECT is one of those inner sections. While mold hurts all systems of the body, some systems require extra protection from the hazards of mold and mold toxins. These areas are:

- Brain and nervous system
- Immune system
- Respiratory system
- Digestive system
- Liver and kidneys
- Skin
- Bladder
- Eyes

My intention with the PROTECT section is to give you a list of tools to choose from. You don't have to do all of these things. I want you to have a well-stocked toolbox My suggestion is to target where you personally are most affected, where you have symptoms.

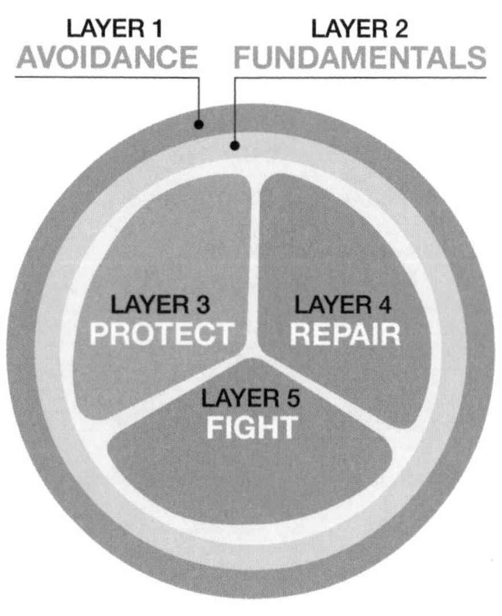

The PROTECT section involves the following...

1 Binders
2 Bile Movers
3 Peloid Therapy
4 DHA
5 Quercetin
6 Milk Thistle
7 Turmeric

1 BINDERS

If you've heard anything about treating mold sickness, you've heard passionate recommendations for binders, meaning bile binders. Why?

Bile carries mold toxins. Think of it as a courier. In the process of normal digestion, bile delivers stuff from the liver to the gut. Like a delivery service, it then returns to the liver to pick up more stuff to drop off in the gut, and on and on the cycle goes.

The problem is that mold toxins are sticky. They won't let go of the bile when it tries to drop them off in the gut. So the bile brings the toxin back to the liver to be reprocessed and repackaged. The liver hands over the package to the bile, who comes back with it again, and again, and again. The definition of detoxification insanity!

Unfortunately, every time the liver or kidneys are presented with mold toxins to be reprocessed, these organs get a little more damaged. Bile binders purposefully interrupt this cycle. The bile gets held up in the gut by the binder and subsequently pooped out. Then we make new, clean bile. Bile binders stop the insanity.

Environmental medicine guru, Dr. Walter Crinnion has been treating environmental illnesses of all kinds for decades, including mold. He uses fibers that have been shown to bind bile and reduce toxin burden. In his book, *Clean, Green, and Lean,* Dr. Crinnion recommends rice bran fiber. Rice bran fiber and other similar fibers work very effectively at grabbing toxin-laden bile from the intestines so they're pooped out and not reabsorbed.

It's wise to add a binding fiber as a supplement if you have mold symptoms. The cool thing about fiber is its regulating action. If you poop too much, it slows things to a normal pace. And if you don't poop enough, it helps with that too.

Fiber also feeds our beneficial gut bacteria, which boosts our gut immune system and aids in nutrient absorption.

Choosing which fiber is right for you is a very individual thing. For mycotoxin binding, find a source high in insoluble fiber. There are plenty of fibers out there, but they don't all grab mold toxins. The list below includes mycotoxin-binding fibers in order of least constipating to most constipating, according to my mold-sick patients. Choose one that doesn't make you go either too much or too little. I find that blends work best. Use only organic sources.

BINDERS

FIBERS TO USE

- **Flax seed**
- **Chia seed**
- **Rice bran**
- **Oat bran**
- **Psyllium husk**

Some people need a stronger intervention.

Pioneering doctor, researcher, and mold warrior, Dr. Ritchie Shoemaker, revolutionized the use of a prescription binder called cholestyramine for mold toxicity. He identified that his patients who were exposed to water-damaged buildings suffered multisystemic, multisymptomatic conditions, which were helped by using cholestyramine.

Cholestyramine works very effectively for mold-sick people by binding toxin-laden bile, so it can be evacuated. It has a higher binding capacity than the fibers listed above, which has some good and some bad aspects. Good: really effective for binding mycotoxins. Bad: can also bind some nutrients and medications, rendering them ineffective. This drug works best taken multiple times per day, and timing the doses gets a little tricky if you also take other medications.

I like to start with fiber and then use the drug cholestyramine if we aren't getting anywhere. I find that if people peel the first two layers of the orange, most have success with the insoluble fibers listed above.

BUT here's my issue with binders.

No Binders If You're Already Bound Up

Many mold-sick patients are constipated. In some people, binders can slow things down and make constipation much worse. This is bad news if you have mycotoxins floating around in your intestines. Lingering mycotoxins damage the surface of your intestinal lining and nuke your gut immune system.

Not everyone does well on binders. Here are some steps toward using binders successfully. It all has to do with how you poo.

BINDERS

HOW TO

STEP 1 If you poop 2-3 times per day, go to Step 4, add fiber.

STEP 2 If you don't have at least one bowel movement a day, start by eating 4 cups of leafy greens every day. If this helps you poo 1-2 times per day, skip to Step 4, add fiber.

STEP 3 Add 1 cup of long grain brown rice to your daily diet.

-If you can still poop regularly, add a fiber supplement per Step 4, and eat the rice when it sounds good.

-If you aren't pooping at least 1 time per day, skip forward to the next section on *Bile Movers*. Once you're pooping 1-2 times per day using bile movers, return to Step 1.

STEP 4 Add an insoluble fiber supplement. Take 1 tablespoon daily with a meal.

STEP 5 Increase fiber to 1 tablespoon two times daily with meals, as long as you're still pooping 1-2 times per day.

STEP 6 As you heal from mold sickness, reduce fiber to 1 tablespoon daily. Watch to make sure you can still go poo regularly. If so, continue a healthy diet and 1 tablespoon of fiber daily to bind up the junk from the dying mold. If you can't poo, stay on the higher dose, and add bile movers if needed. (see the next section)

STEP 7 When the mold treatment is done, continue a healthy diet and use fiber only as needed. If you aren't pooping at least 2 times per day, stay on the fiber supplement.

BINDERS
CAUTIONS

Constipation: Make sure to have a minimum of 2 bowel movements daily while taking any fiber product during mold treatment. If not, use bile movers. You must be pooping to get better.

Medication timing: If you take medications, check whether any medication needs to be taken away from fiber supplements.

Fungal overgrowth: Some people with fungal overgrowth get uncomfortable bloating from eating any grain, even high fiber rice. If this is you, skip Step 3 above.

Medications: With some classes of anticoagulant drugs relating to vitamin K, patients are told not to eat green vegetables. That's crazy. We need our greens for all the other parts of our bodies.

Adjust the medication around the greens in your diet, BUT be prescriptive about eating daily greens or take a greens powder supplement. Do not miss.

2 BILE MOVERS

I would much rather a mold-sick person have diarrhea than constipation. We want toxins released from dying mold to be flushed rather than absorbed. We achieve that by using bile moving agents.

Laxatives don't help a mold-sick person as much as bile movers, but both have the same effect in the end. Bile stimulates the bowels like laxatives do, but it also grabs mold toxins. There are a host of things to choose from in this category. For mold, I use herbs called cholagogues, and supplements called bile salts.

Cholagogues are the first place to start. These bitter tasting plants and herbs induce bile secretion. Tasting the flavor of bitter makes mold toxins available for binding. I encourage everyone to incorporate bitter greens into their diets. Work your way into it; bitter can be an acquired taste.

Try bitter greens such as arugula, broccoli rabe, endive, watercress, kale, or dandelion greens. Green tea is considered a bitter and contains mold-protective bioflavonoids. In moderation, add a little dark chocolate or coffee, but notice I said a little.

If you have mold symptoms, can't poop, and adding bitters to your diet didn't help, you'll need something stronger. You'll need medicinal bitter herbs—cholagogues.

Cholagogue herbs work best if you taste them. I recommend putting drops of tincture of cholagogues directly on the tongue for maximal bile-moving effect. A lovely, palatable blend that's both bitter and sweet is called Sweetish Bitters.

If the taste is too strong, and you simply can't bring yourself to that level of commitment, you can take them in a pill form. But I recommend opening one capsule into the bottle and shaking it around to coat the outside of the capsule so your taste buds get a tiny hint.

Bile salts are used for those with gall bladder insufficiency. Some mold-sick people have defective gall bladders. They may have been born that way. In my training, they're called nonsecretors because they don't make robust digestive juices, including bile. This group tends to be more susceptible to environmental toxin-based illnesses. Check out Dr. Peter D'Adamo's book *Eat Right 4 Your Type* for more information.

Some mold-sick people have defective gall bladders because their gall bladders are overloaded with gunky mold toxins. The gall bladder can no longer squeeze out bile when they eat. These people may need to include bile salts with every meal.

If you can't poop, I recommend using cholagogue herbs with each meal. If still no action, add bile salts to every meal. And then, only if you can poop 1-2 times per day, add a toxin-binding fiber. Often, once the mold population gets knocked back, and your body gains strength, you won't need as much of a push.

BILE MOVERS

HOW TO

CHOLAGOGUE

Try First: Eat bitter greens with each meal. If not pooping regularly, add tincture of bitters.

Add: Add tincture of bitters by taking 5 drops directly on the tongue, 10 minutes before each meal.

Add If Needed: Add 1 capsule of cholagogue herbs, such as dandelion root, red root, gentian, or chelidonium. Ask your doctor which one is right for your constitution.

BILE SALTS

Look for organic supplements that say "bile salts" or "ox bile". Take 1 supplement with your largest 2 meals daily if adding cholagogues hasn't given you the bowel relief you're looking for.

BILE MOVERS

CAUTIONS

This is a level of complexity that will probably require a mold-literate doctor.

Diarrhea: Bile movers can cause diarrhea.

Gall stones: Proceed slowly and cautiously if you have gall bladder problems. If you have gall stones, moving bile may cause a gall bladder attack and rarely, induce your gall bladder to expel stones.

3 PELOID THERAPY

Peloid is basically a fancy word for mud bath. But this isn't any old mud. Peloids use peat mud. I refer to this therapy as "sneaky peat," because the beneficial effects sneak up on you. It doesn't feel like you've done anything. You just sat in dirty bath water. Yet you get profound results. It seems too easy to be that good.

Peloid therapies have been used throughout the ages for a variety of health complaints. Peloids, or peat mud applications, boost our skin's ability to expel toxins. In the case of mold, it's a real champ.

I find that some people's bodies are so loaded with mold toxin, their bodies have lost the ability to get rid of the garbage, even after leaving the sick environment. Their emunctories are too full to keep moving, and the backup of toxin causes symptoms. That's when you call for the help of sneaky peat. I like to use this method with mold-sick people who suffer from constipation, sinus congestion, lymphatic stagnation, cellulite, and skin issues.

Remember the hockey player with the rashes? Soaking in peat mud baths was critical to clearing up his skin. Because his skin was the main source of the mycotoxin exposure, his skin and the layers below were overloaded. They had soaked up mycotoxins from his pads and stored them.

Peloids are easy to do at home.

PELOID THERAPY

HOW TO

Hydrate excessively ahead of time with spring water.

STEP 1 Fill a bathtub with comfortably hot water. Caution, the water may heat up once the mud is added, so don't go too crazy with the hot water.

STEP 2 Add one container of Moor Mud soak (see *Resources* section for source).

STEP 3 Soak in the tub for 25-40 minutes. For your first bath, soak for only 25 minutes to test your body's reaction.

STEP 4 When finished soaking, drain the tub and lightly rinse off the mud.

STEP 5 Without drying off, wrap in a warm blanket, and lie down for 30-45 minutes. It's common to feel like your inner temperature rises, and to sweat more than you have in a long time.

STEP 6 After 30-45 minutes, rinse off thoroughly with a cool shower.

STEP 7 Hydrate again.

PELOID THERAPY

CAUTION

Open wounds: Be cautious if you have open wounds to make sure they aren't getting irritated or infected.

High blood pressure: If you have high blood pressure, start with less time. Test with a shorter time frame in the mud soak to make sure your blood pressure can remain stable during the soak, and at 1 hour following the soak.

4 DHA

DHA stands for decosahexanoic acid. Yeah, let's just stick with DHA. DHA is a beneficial dietary fat that comes primarily from fish. DHA protects the brain, nervous system, and eyes.

Mold can really affect how your brain works; symptoms such as foggy mind, slowed thinking, confusion, difficulty finding the right word, brain fatigue, and even dementia. A large part of this is DHA deficiency. Dementia specialist, Dr. Dale Bredesen, refers to mold-brain as Inhalational Alzheimer's disease, a subtype of Alzheimer's disease. He's leading the charge to make people aware that Inhalational Alzheimer's is a treatable disease. See more in the *Resources* section.

Many of my mold-sick patients complain of vision changes since their exposure. This is due to both direct eye damage and damage to the visual processing part of the brain. DHA helps both targets.

DHA also restores the function of your mitochondria—the powerhouse of your cells. Mold-sick people who are low in DHA feel like they have aged many years older than their actual age.

If mold is mostly affecting your brain, energy, nerves, or eyes, DHA is your friend.

DHA

HOW TO

Food: Eat clean fish four days per week. Check out the Environmental Working Group's list of mercury-free fish choices.

Supplement: 3 grams daily of DHA. As your neurological symptoms improve, wean down slowly and get what you need via diet.

In studies, up to 30 grams were safely taken during acute exposure events.

DHA

CAUTIONS

Fish allergy: Avoid DHA if you have an allergy to fish. Close plant-based substitutes are borage oil, primrose oil, and black currant oil.

Bleeding risk: There's a theoretical issue when combining DHA with anticoagulant drugs. This is still to be proven in studies, but keep an eye out for easy bruising if you take an anticoagulant medication.

5 QUERCETIN

Quercetin is a bioflavonoid, which means it's colorful. The colorful part of plants are the most beneficial for mold recovery. Quercetin has an affinity for the sinuses, gut, and bladder. It's an anti-inflammatory. It actually rewires your propensity to be inflamed when exposed to allergens. People who develop allergies after mold exposure love this neon yellow pigment. They say that if it weren't for Quercetin, their eyes would be swollen shut and their bellies would be in pain. Quercetin comes from the skins of onions. Isn't that ironic? Quercetin heals the runny eyes, drippy nose, and indigestion that onions can cause raw.

QUERCETIN

HOW TO

Food: Eat onions. I'm a big fan of Julia Child's original recipe for French Onion soup. It's divine! And when you have mold sickness, it's the only thing to hit the spot some days.

Supplement: Take 300-600mg capsules, from 1 to 3 times daily.

QUERCETIN

CAUTIONS

This is a very safe supplement.

Nose bleeds: I've rarely seen excessive use of Quercetin dry the respiratory passages so much that it caused nosebleeds from dryness. This was only in patients that were still exposed to their moldy environments.

6 MILK THISTLE

Milk thistle is a champion for mold recovery. It protects our vital organs, the liver and kidneys. These organs take a direct hit from the toxins secreted by mold. There are even liver cancers directly linked to certain mycotoxin exposures. If you have symptoms involving the liver and/or the kidneys, milk thistle must be part of your regimen.

You might be wondering what liver or kidney symptoms look like. Think chemical sensitivity, acute sense of smell, visual floaters, headaches, nausea after eating, abdominal bloating, wimpy appetite, alcohol cravings, swollen hands and feet, increase in age spots, low back pain, strong smelling urine, or low urine output. These are just a few of the vague symptoms connected to liver and kidney strain.

It turns out, milk thistle not only protects, but can also correct long-term effects from mold. Put literally, it regenerates new liver cells. That's a medical miracle! These effects weren't seen at low doses. You need a minimum daily dose to reach the basic protective effects. With milk thistle, dose matters, and so does organic sourcing.

MILK THISTLE

HOW TO

Minimum daily dose: Take 750mg of organic milk thistle seed powder (Silybum marinum) daily.

Milk thistle is safely taken up to 1500mg daily to rid the body of the toxic effects of mold.

If you've gotten quite sick from mold exposure, this is one supplement to remain on long-term. As mold dies, it can spill more mycotoxins. You don't want to be left unprotected.

MILK THISTLE
CAUTIONS

Drug interactions: Medications that are processed through the cytochrome p450 system in the liver may interact with this herb. Ask your doctor if your medication is in this category. Often a simple dose adjustment can be made.

7 TURMERIC

Turmeric is known for a multitude of benefits in the body, but for mold, it truly shines. Remember that mold affects many body systems? Well so does turmeric, but in a good way. It's an antioxidant, protects the liver and kidneys, and can help the body at the gene level to boost glutathione, the chief antioxidant.

It would be hard for me to narrow down a symptom list for turmeric since it helps so many areas. But if I had to choose, I'd say brain function, inflammatory pain, neurogenic pain, and all the liver stuff listed above in the *Milk Thistle* section.

I recommend starting at very small doses at first. If you don't eat curry regularly, start there. Some people with a lot of toxic buildup can feel worse if they take too much of this herb because it starts the detox process with fervor. The most common negative reaction is headache. If you've peeled the outer layers of the orange first, this is usually not a problem.

Turmeric is absorbed best when simmered with oils or processed specifically to be fat-soluble. Seek brands that have taken this extra processing step, and use only organic sources. Don't skimp on cost. Poorly made turmeric supplements go in the front door and out the back without stopping.

TURMERIC

HOW TO

Food: For 5 days in a row, eat curry containing 1 teaspoon turmeric powder that's been simmered in oil. Coconut oil is a nice option.

Supplement: If you don't have any negative reactions to dietary turmeric, take 350mg liposomal turmeric (Curcuma longa).

If you tolerate it alright, it's safely taken up to 350mg, three times daily.

TURMERIC

CAUTIONS

Drug interactions: Like milk thistle, medications that are processed through the cytochrome p450 system in the liver may interact with this herb. Ask your doctor if your medication is in this category. Often a simple dose adjustment can be made.

2.4 Repair

You may wonder why I've dedicated an entire chapter to REPAIR. I liken being exposed to mold as being hit by a heat-seeking bomb. Mold not only destroys normal body functions but also seems to seek out areas of the body that could repair the damage and wrecks them too. The largest aspect of REPAIR is to first remove the mycotoxins and then repair the wreckage they left behind.

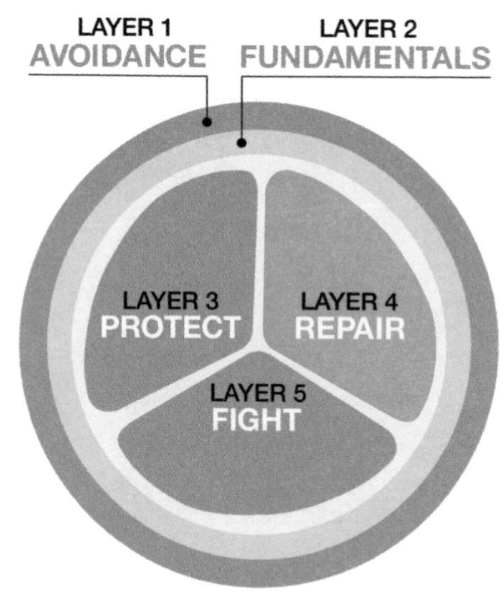

DAMAGE FROM MYCOTOXINS TO REPAIR

Mycotoxins are the most harmful aspects of mold exposure. They can be poisoning us without any trace or scent. These are the negative effects of mycotoxins that require REPAIR:

- Neurotoxicity to the brain and nerves
- Immune depletion
- Destruction of linings of digestion and bladder
- Liver dysfunction, specifically glutathione depletion
- Kidney damage
- Heart muscle and conduction effects
- Skin toxicity
- Reprogramming genes to lower your defenses
- Increased aging via oxidative damage

You've peeled the orange, and chosen select tools to PROTECT. Now pick a tool or two to help REPAIR. Of all the things below, make sure to support glutathione if your doctor has found mycotoxins on your tests.

REPAIR tools to choose from...

1 Lymphatic massage
2 Sauna
3 Bioflavonoids
4 Resveratrol
5 Glutathione
6 Alpha-lipoic acid
7 Melatonin
8 Coenzyme Q10

1 LYMPHATIC MASSAGE

Remember that the lymph system is our body's sanitation system. The lymph channels are the sewer lines, and our organs of detoxification package that waste to be pooped out of the body. Lymphatic congestion and toxicity is a major problem with mold-sick people.

Symptoms of lymphatic congestion are mottled appearance to the skin, cellulite, skin rashes, swollen or chronically hardened lymph nodes, winded after moving your body, swelling of gravity-dependent limbs, headache, congested ears, achy groin, bounding pulse after eating, full and doughy abdomen, and frequent infections. For this, I recommend lymphatic massage.

Lymphatic massage is different from a regular massage. There's no trigger point digging or deep tissue muscle work. To target the lymph, the practitioner puts only enough pressure to hold a nickel against a wall without it dropping. It's very, very light pressure. It's hard for our minds to comprehend this.

I've made the mistake of forgetting to warn patients of this difference. I referred them for lymphatic massage without describing it and got complaint calls. They felt like they had wasted their money because there was no deep tissue work. Well, that's not the point of a lymphatic massage. The point is to move lymph channels just under the skin layer. You may feel cruddy after your first one because of all the toxins that got moved around.

LYMPHATIC MASSAGE
HOW TO

Schedule specifically with a lymphatic massage therapist. Ask to see proof of their training. Terms to look for are lymphedema, lymphatic edema or lymphatic drainage. Cancer centers are good resources to find a trained practitioner.

Start with one lymphatic massage and see how you feel.

If you didn't feel any reaction at all, you don't need this intervention.

If you did have a reaction of any kind, keep going until you don't.

LYMPHATIC MASSAGE

CAUTIONS

Headache: This is usually due to dehydration and/or low glutathione status. Make sure you're hydrated with good quality spring water. If that doesn't help, reference the *Glutathione* section.

Kidney disease: If you have kidney disease, the amount of lymph movement can cause fluid overload and stress your kidneys. The problem is, if you have kidney disease, you need this intervention more than anyone else. I recommend scheduling short, frequent, single-limb focused lymphatic massages to work with your kidney challenges but still get the positive effects.

2 SAUNA

Saunas have been used for hundreds of years for detoxification. Research suggests that it's not so much what you sweat out but that you moved blood around. Like a radiator, blood circulates from your core to your skin to cool you from the sauna's heat. This blood pumping action picks up toxins along the way and brings them back to your organs of detoxification. There they get packaged in bile to be evacuated.

Because it's not just "the sweat," but rather the movement of blood, sauna is the perfect agent for those too sick to exercise, just like we talked about in the FUNDAMENTALS section. Yes, you need water in, and water out, but you must also move it around. Sauna accomplishes this feat. Remember, once you are well enough to move, also move your body. It's still the best.

Mold treatment innovator and educator, Dr. Joseph Brewer, shared a case example of a patient who was using far-infrared sauna therapy as part of her treatment plan. Her urine mycotoxins increased ten-fold after the sauna. This result further supports the theory that detoxification is increased by moving blood around. I've seen exercise have the same effect.

SAUNA

HOW TO

Traditional dry-heat sauna: 150-175 °F (75-100 °C) for 30-45 minutes. Rinse immediately after stepping out with as cold a shower as you can stand for 1 minute, no longer. Northerners can jump in a snow bank.

Far-infrared sauna: 125-130 °F (52-55 °C) for 25-30 minutes. More sweating often occurs after you leave the sauna. Enhance this by wrapping up in a warm blanket until sweating stops, and then rinse with a cool shower.

SAUNA

CAUTIONS

Dehydration: Dehydration is the most common problem for people using sauna therapy. For the 4 hours prior to using a sauna, hydrate with spring water at a rate of 6 ounces or more per half hour.

High blood pressure: If you have high blood pressure, monitor your blood pressure during the sauna. I like wrist blood pressure monitors due to ease of use and lack of restriction of lymph flow.

Kidney disease: Sauna can challenge the kidneys' ability to filter blood and make urine. If you have kidney disease, your doctor may want you to monitor your urine specific gravity before, during, and after sauna. Start with half the time recommended to make sure your kidneys can manage the challenge.

3 BIOFLAVONOIDS

Bioflavonoids are your color-guard. They're the colorful pigments in vegetables and fruits. Bioflavonoids are incredibly powerful at protecting you from the negative effects of mold spores and toxins. They protect and prevent damage all the way down to the cell level. If you have long-standing mold problems that are affecting you with Category 2 or 3 symptoms on the Crista Mold Questionnaire, you need a food intervention.

The best way to get bioflavonoids is by eating them. There's a certain mold-fighting branch of that family, called polyphenols. Green tea and matcha green tea are very high in polyphenols and have powerful mold healing properties. Another pigment, a red one called lycopene, helps with mycotoxin repair. Lycopene is high in tomatoes. The yellow pigment, called Quercetin, is so helpful for mold, it got its own section in the book. Greens, reds, yellows, purples…as you see, it takes the whole rainbow of colors.

BIOFLAVONOIDS

HOW TO

Food: Eat 5-7 servings of a rainbow of colors of vegetables every day.

Food: Eat 1-2 servings of a rainbow of colors of fruits every day IF you don't have fungal overgrowth.

Drink: 2 cups of green tea daily. If you don't care for green tea, add 1/2 teaspoon of matcha green tea to your food. Or drink chamomile tea. Chamomile repairs mycotoxin damage and tastes sweet with an ever-so-soft amount of bitter.

BIOFLAVONOIDS

CAUTIONS

Organic: Don't make your toxicity problem worse by eating toxic vegetables. Check out the Environmental Working Group's Dirty Dozen and Clean Thirteen lists. Use these handy references to guide your organic buying. You can either pay for organic food or doctor visits, your choice.

Weight loss: If mold-sickness has caused you to lose too much weight, you may need fewer servings of plants and more proteins and fats. Eating this many organic vegetables will usually induce fat loss via toxin loss. Monitor your weight.

Medications: With some classes of anticoagulant drugs relating to vitamin K, patients are told not to eat green vegetables. That's crazy. We need our greens for all the other parts of our bodies.

Adjust the medication around the greens in your diet, BUT be prescriptive about eating daily greens or take a greens powder supplement. Do not miss.

4 RESVERATROL

Resveratrol is a potent antioxidant. It repairs damage to the liver and the nervous system, and it has anticancer properties after mycotoxin exposure. It's gotten a lot of press as the excuse to drink red wine. It's true, red wine contains resveratrol, but to get the amount of resveratrol required to combat the effects of mold, you'd have to drink 60 bottles of red wine every day. No, I didn't just recommend drinking 60 bottles of red wine…not even 1 bottle of red wine every day.

I have concerns about red wine. As we learned in the case about the woman who increasingly developed food sensitivities, red wine can contain mycotoxins. If you do enjoy a bit of red wine with your meals, make sure the winemaker provides independent tests for mycotoxins. There are wine buying clubs that make this search easier (see the *Resources* section).

Big picture, this one needs to be supplemented. Resveratrol helps with generalized aches and pains, low energy, skin problems, and sluggish circulation, and it may lower cholesterol. It's touted as an age defier. Research shows the benefits of resveratrol were seen if participants maintained a daily minimum dose of 1 gram (1000 mg) daily.

RESVERATROL
HOW TO

Supplement: Ingest a minimum of 1000mg daily. After a few months killing mold (FIGHT section), try cutting the dose in half. Watch over the next week to make sure you still feel well. If not, go back up to 1000mg daily, and try to wean yourself off at a later date.

CAUTIONS

Non-fermented sources: Japanese knotweed is the most common plant source for resveratrol. Many herbal processors access the resveratrol by fermenting Japanese knotweed. There's nothing wrong with that for normal people, but mold exposed people often have a bad reaction. Even though there aren't any fungal (mold) elements left in the resveratrol after processing, simply having been fermented can pose a problem. See the *Resources* section for companies that use extraction versus fermentation.

5 GLUTATHIONE

Glutathione is the single most powerful antioxidant against mycotoxins. Boom!

> All Mycotoxins
> **Deplete Glutathione**

Glutathione is king. If you're a Lord of the Rings fan, you'll understand my label for glutathione. I call it "the one antioxidant to rule them all." In fairness, vitamin C could also take this title for general purposes, but when it comes to mold, glutathione wins.

Yes, all mycotoxins deplete glutathione. Low glutathione levels leads to dysfunction of basic metabolic processes at our very core, at the DNA level. Without glutathione, we become toxic waste dumps. The liver, kidneys, brain, lungs, and immune system limp along trying to deal with all the garbage. That's where symptoms come in.

Glutathione eases symptoms in the brain and nervous system, the respiratory system, and organs of detoxification—primarily the liver, but also the kidneys.

Form matters. The best way to get glutathione into the body is intravenously. It's hard to find a doctor who offers IV glutathione. If you are lucky enough to live somewhere with this resource, well done you. The rest of us need to take it as a supplement. I recommend using only liposomal forms. I've had mixed results and have landed on a few favorites based on reliable clinical outcomes and improved lab tests (see the *Resources* section). Before using glutathione, take an extra step to make sure you aren't allergic to it.

GLUTATHIONE
HOW TO

STEP 1 Moisten a cotton swab with a small amount of the liquid liposomal glutathione and swipe inside the cheek or nose. If you have a localized reaction, you may have sulfite sensitivity and can't use glutathione. Use milk thistle and selenium to boost your body's ability to make its own glutathione as an alternative.

STEP 2 If no reaction, take 225mg of oral liposomal liquid glutathione early in the day. Watch for new or worsening symptoms. If they develop, cut the dose in half and try again. If that doesn't even work, make sure you go back to the FUNDAMENTALS section and work on Emunctories.

STEP 3 After 1 week, if you didn't develop worsening or new symptoms, take 450mg of oral liposomal liquid glutathione daily, early in the day.

STEP 4 Monitor lab values to determine how long to stay on glutathione.

STEP 5 If you've been taking glutathione for a long time and can't seem to keep your levels up without supplementation, you may be deficient in selenium. Selenium is easy to supplement and has its own mycotoxin repair properties. You may also need genetic support. See the *Resources* section for Dr. Benjamin Lynch's book, *Dirty Genes*.

GLUTATHIONE

CAUTIONS

Taste: Warning! Glutathione tastes like liquid farts. For real. It's terrible. Orange juice can usually mask the farty flavor well enough to get it down. If your glutathione doesn't taste terrible, I'm suspect of its potency. There are other forms available: transdermal, intranasal, and nebulized. I don't have much experience monitoring lab values with these, so I can't comment on their efficacy.

Detox reactions: If you've been sick from mold a long time, chances are you've been low on glutathione a long time. If so, you may have a few days of feeling like you've been hit by a truck once you start adding back this powerful antioxidant. This should only last 2-3 days at the most. If this feeling lasts longer, temporarily stop glutathione and follow the Herx tools in the FIGHT section.

Sulfite sensitivity: People with sulfite sensitivity tend not to tolerate glutathione.

Asthmatics: Nebulized glutathione may make asthma worse during a flare.

6 ALPHA-LIPOIC ACID

Alpha-lipoic acid (ALA) is a precursor to glutathione. Some people who can't tolerate glutathione do very well on ALA. It has most of the same beneficial effects of protecting the liver and kidneys, but adds a little magic of its own. ALA reduces inflammation and protects the immune system at the gene level. It also can stabilize blood sugar.

If you find that you get sick all the time, that colds linger or go to your lungs, or if you have unstable blood sugar, ALA is a good match.

ALPHA-LIPOIC ACID
HOW TO

Supplement: Take 600mg Alpha-lipoic acid (ALA) capsules 2 times daily.

ALPHA-LIPOIC ACID
CAUTIONS

Sulfite sensitivity: For more direction for what to do if you're sensitive to sulfites, check out Dr. BenjaminLynch's book, *Dirty Genes*.

7 MELATONIN

I stated before that the single most powerful mold antioxidant was glutathione, and this is true. But melatonin is the single most powerful *brain* antioxidant against mold and mycotoxins. Melatonin helps "mold-brain," that foggy sense like you're losing your edge. As melatonin heals brain tissue, "mold-brain" symptoms improve.

Melatonin also repairs damage to the liver and kidneys. In the liver, melatonin repairs liver cells that have been injured so badly, they otherwise would die off. Melatonin also stimulates the liver to make its own glutathione.

If your primary symptoms are liver symptoms, melatonin will be your liver's friend. This is a nice supplement to use in combination with *milk thistle*. Liver symptoms pulled from the list in the Milk Thistle section are chemical sensitivity, acute sense of smell, visual floaters, headaches, nausea after eating, abdominal bloating, wimpy appetite, alcohol cravings, swollen hands and feet, and increase in age spots. These are just a few of the vague symptoms connected to liver damage.

To achieve the desired brain and liver effects, we follow doses established by cancer therapy. Even though 1-3mg of melatonin helps you fall asleep, we dose much higher for mold repair.

Higher doses won't usually help you fall asleep, so you have to make sure to induce your own. Melatonin's mold repairing effects are amplified if combined with CoQ10 (as described in the next section).

MELATONIN

HOW TO

Induce Your Own Melatonin: Help induce your own natural melatonin by using very little lighting for the hour before bedtime. Melatonin is strongest if you follow the sun's timing. The worst thing for natural melatonin production is screen time within the two hours before bedtime. Join my crusade to go to sleep when the sun goes down! If we all do it, the night owls won't have anyone to talk to, and they might fall asleep too.

Supplement: Take 20mg before bed daily.

MELATONIN

CAUTIONS

Dreams: While it won't necessarily help you sleep at high doses, some patients reported strange dreams for the first few weeks after starting melatonin.

Drowsiness: We give melatonin at night just in case it makes you sleepy.

8 **COENZYME Q10** (CoQ10)

Okay, where I stated before that the single most powerful mold antioxidant was glutathione, I really meant it. But next to melatonin being the single most powerful brain antioxidant against mycotoxins, CoQ10 is the single most powerful *heart* antioxidant. You might be noticing a trend that antioxidants are good for mold treatment, and that I get excited about them.

People with sustained exposure to certain mycotoxins can get damage to their heart muscle, called myocarditis. This is caused by inflammation and a mold-induced CoQ10 deficiency in the heart muscle cells. CoQ10 feeds the mitochondria, or powerhouses, of the heart muscle cells. These guys can't take a day off. They can't even take a second off...or our hearts would stop.

If you've been experiencing heart symptoms or chest discomfort in conjunction with your other mold symptoms, it could be CoQ10 deficiency. Get your heart looked at by your doctor. Not everything is mold. If everything cardiovascularly checks out, adding CoQ10 can give you relief, and increase your overall energy.

CoQ10 helps other areas of your body affected by mold, like skeletal muscles. For example, some people say they feel wiped out whenever they try to exert themselves. That's the mitochondria running out of gas. CoQ10 feeds them.

And as mentioned above, CoQ10 also heals the liver and kidneys, especially when combined with melatonin.

Look for CoQ10 supplements that are in the form of dissolvable chews. Resist the temptation to chew them. The longer they take to dissolve, the more CoQ10 you've absorbed right through your cheeks.

COENZYME Q10

HOW TO

STEP 1 Most people get relief taking 100mg daily.

STEP 2 If you're having chest-related symptoms, take 100mg three times daily.

STEP 3 As symptoms ease, drop to 2 times daily and watch how you do under exertion. If your chest-related symptoms come back, go back up to 3 times daily. Try reducing at a later date, after you've killed more mold from your body.

COENZYME Q10

CAUTIONS

Allergy: Rarely, patients have reported allergies to CoQ10. In my practice, it was the flavorants in the tablet, not the CoQ10. They tolerated the pill form just fine.

2.5
Fight

It's finally time to BREAK THE MOLD.

Okay, you've mastered AVOIDANCE, you have the FUNDAMENTALS in place, and you've added selective tools to PROTECT your body and REPAIR damage from the exposure. You're ready. But so is mold.

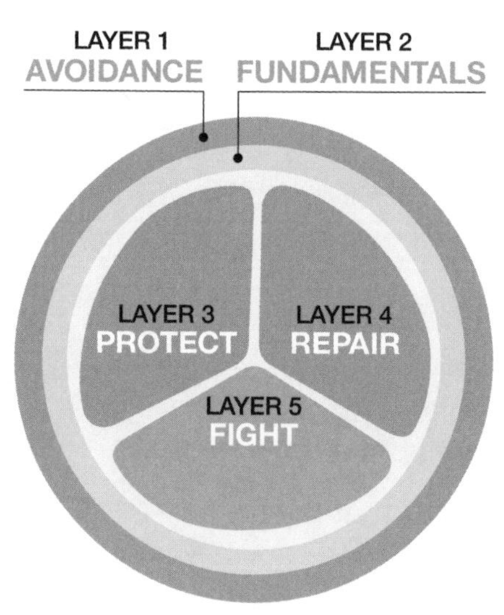

Killing mold is sort of like trying to clean a bear cage while the bear is still inside. You wait until it falls asleep, then tiptoe in to mop up the place, as quietly as possible with the least disruption… and you never, ever "poke the bear."

I've seen in practice that once mold knows it's the target of your assault, it will dig in its heels and try to defend its territory, which it has now claimed as YOU. I've seen reactions such as raging sweet cravings, digestive bloating, terrible ear ringing, sleep problems for nights on end, and worsening fungal infections, to name a few. Stick to it as long as it's not too hard. These are temporary annoyances. I know, they may be extremely annoying, but they mean you're on the right track. Don't be afraid to seek medical help from your doctor during the Fight phase, as you may need a little extra help.

These are the aspects of the FIGHT tool...

Whole-body antifungals

1 Pau D'Arco
2 Holy Basil
3 Olive Leaf
4 Old Man's Beard
5 Thyme
6 Oil of Oregano

Nasal antifungals

7 Essential oils
8 Colloidal silver
9 Ozone
10 Xylitol

Finish the job

11 Biofilm busters
12 Herx helpers
13 Reintroduction

GO ON THE OFFENSIVE

It's said that the best defense is a strong offense—totally true in mold sickness. To rid yourself of mold inhabitation, you have to make your body completely inhospitable. You have to kill mold two ways: whole-body and nasal. Nasal antifungals are targeted treatments that knock out the colonies residing in your sinuses. Whereas, whole-body antifungals clean up the gut and kill any mold that scatters when you hit the sinuses with your offensive. It's best to have whole-body antifungals on board before beginning any nasal treatment.

Herbs are incredible allies for this. Prescription antifungal medications usually have only one or two ways to hit mold. Not so for herbs. A single antifungal herb has many, many different weapons to kill mold. Not only does this make herbs effective mold killers, it also reduces mold's ability to revive itself.

> **To Win Against Mold,** Use Whole-Body AND Nasal Antifungals
>
> **Don't Use One Without The Other**

Mold is smart. If you only have one weapon, it'll find a work-around to survive despite the treatment. This is called resistance. If antifungal drugs are needed, they can be combined with select herbs for a full assault, with the added benefit of reduced drug resistance.

Herbs usually also contain compounds that reduce side effects from dying mold. Many antifungal herbs kill mold and clean up mycotoxin spillage, and protect the liver, and repair the gut, and so on. I like using herbs because they have a low harm ratio compared to their efficacy.

WHOLE-BODY ANTIFUNGALS

To fully recover, treat your whole body with antifungal therapies. The people who don't get better leave this piece out. Even though they've left the sick environment and completed nasal treatment, the mold comes back.

There's a misconception that you have to have an active fungal infection in order to take these herbs. False. The truth is that even though colonization is not infection, mold colonies continuously seed mold spores and spit out mycotoxins. You can be sick from mold without having a fungal infection. And if you're sick from mold, you need antifungals for your whole body so those spores don't find a place to take root.

How long do you take whole-body antifungals? Until you are sure there are no more mycotoxins in your system—plus one more month for insurance. Mycotoxins come from mold spores. If you've killed all the mold spores and detoxed the mycotoxins, there shouldn't be any more mycotoxins on your labs. If there are, you either didn't do AVOIDANCE fully, or there's still surviving mold somewhere inside your body.

The plants I discuss are safe enough to take long-term. For instance, Pau D'Arco and Holy Basil are enjoyed as morning tea in many cultures. With my patients, I rotate herbs every month or so to make sure mold isn't figuring out a work-around. This also ensures that we aren't taxing the body or creating nutritional deficiencies.

I've listed treatments in order of intensity and potential to create side effects, from least to most. Don't mistake intensity with efficacy. Intensity has to do with the other actions a plant has that are not related to mold. The least-intense plants can kill more mold by being able to be taken more frequently.

You're in this for the long haul. Often I will use something less intense continuously and do bursts of more intense plants for shorter durations, for example, daily Pau D'Arco tea with bursts of Oil of Oregano three days per week. This is where the art of medicine comes in. Again, I recommend seeing a mold-literate doctor to discern what to do and when.

Fantastic whole-body antifungal herbs include:

1. Pau D'Arco
2. Holy Basil
3. Olive Leaf
4. Old Man's Beard
5. Thyme
6. Oil of Oregano

1 PAU D'ARCO

Pau D'Arco was used traditionally as a tea by pre-Incas in the rainforests of Central and South America. It's made from the inner bark of the lapacho tree and is known there as taheebo tea. It was used to ward off fungal infections of the respiratory system and skin, which can come from living in continuously warm, moist environments. It's been shown to both protect from fungal spore invasion and treat established fungal infections.

In studies, Pau D'Arco's fungal-killing strength is right up there with powerful antifungal medications, such as amphotericin B, yet it's gentle to the user. It also has broad antimicrobial activity, which is helpful for disrupting established biofilm colonies.

Pau D'Arco loosens deeply embedded mucous. It's especially useful for asthmatics who have trouble clearing their lungs and chronic sinus sufferers. Drinking this tea before bed helps people who get sinus congestion as soon as they lie down. Pau D'Arco builds back the immune system's fortitude and even has anticancer properties.

PAU D'ARCO
HOW TO

Tea: To make your own Pau D'Arco tea, simmer 1 tablespoon of shredded inner bark in 2-3 cups of simmering water, covered, for 10 minutes. Strain, let cool to a comfortable temperature, and drink.

Enjoy this tea several times a day.

Frontier Herbs offers Pau D'Arco in bulk.

Traditional Medicinals makes this in pre-packaged tea bags.

PAU D'ARCO

CAUTIONS

Pregnancy: Do not use Pau D'Arco during pregnancy.

Taste: Pau D'Arco tea has a musky flavor. It can be taken by capsule if taste is a barrier.

2 HOLY BASIL

Holy Basil, or Tulsi as it's known in India, is revered for its health-promoting properties. It is said to have the ability to lighten the mind. Holy Basil is taken traditionally as a tea in Ayurvedic medicine for infections from molds, fungi, bacteria, and parasites. Like Pau A'arco, it has a powerful microbial killing ability while being gentle on the user. If antifungal drugs are needed, Holy Basil is used safely in combination to prevent drug resistance.

I've been lucky enough to learn from Dr. Tieraona Lowdog, who teaches that Holy Basil has an affinity for the lungs. I combine it with Pau D'Arco for patients who developed asthma from exposure to mold. As a mycotoxin detox agent, it's especially useful for those whose heavy mycotoxin burden has dulled the mind.

HOLY BASIL

HOW TO

STEP 1 Steep 1 tablespoon of Holy Basil in 2-3 cups of hot water for up to 5 minutes.

STEP 2 Slowly inhale the fumes while the tea steeps bringing potent essential oils deep into the sinuses and lungs.

STEP 3 Drink several times daily.

Tulsi tea by Organic India comes prepackaged with other mold helpers—Holy Basil with green tea and pomegranate—to make many tools in one.

HOLY BASIL

CAUTIONS

Sleep: Holy Basil may be stimulating to the mind. If this happens to you, avoid it before bedtime.

Taste: Holy Basil is very aromatic. It can be taken by capsule if the taste is a barrier.

3 OLIVE LEAF

Olive Leaf is an antifungal that protects against the invasion of mold by boosting your own immune fighters. This provides a secondary benefit against viruses. By restoring your innate immune system, Olive Leaf can both kill mold and help beat chronic viral infections, such as Epstein-Barr or other herpes family viruses. Mycotoxin exposure makes us more susceptible to these types of viral infections.

Olive Leaf is a handy plant remedy for those with digestive symptoms. It protects the gastrointestinal lining from the damaging effects of mycotoxins. Many people who developed food sensitivities after mold exposure have been able to eat those foods again with the help of Olive Leaf. It can also stabilize blood sugar and reduce cravings for sweets.

OLIVE LEAF

HOW TO

Supplement: A typical dose of Olive Leaf is 500mg of whole plant or extract, taken two times daily. Safe to use long-term.

OLIVE LEAF

CAUTIONS

Indigestion: While rare, Olive Leaf can cause stomach irritation or diarrhea. I find that this occurs if mold-promoting foods are not avoided.

Low blood pressure: One of the benefits of Olive Leaf is that it can lower blood pressure. If you struggle with low blood pressure, watch your blood pressure when taking Olive Leaf. If you get dizzy standing up from sitting, Olive Leaf may not be a sound remedy for you.

Low blood sugar: Monitor your blood sugar to prevent hypoglycemia while taking Olive Leaf.

4 OLD MAN'S BEARD

Old Man's Beard, or Usnea, is named for its appearance. As it hangs in trees, it looks like a scraggly old beard. I was taught that the Native American name translates to "sniffly drippy." I find this to be a useful description of the symptoms it helps. I use Old Man's Beard for mold sufferers with hay fever, allergies, frequent sniffing or sneezing, and chronic sore throat. Old Man's Beard is a sinus allergy sufferer's friend, especially during a cold.

Old Man's Beard is helpful to prevent skin issues from becoming fungal infections, including jock itch and vaginal yeast infections. It inhibits biofilm formation, and it has a particular affinity for the bladder, aiding irritable bladder symptoms when due to mold exposure and mycotoxins.

Old Man's Beard can be tough on the liver, so it should only be used in short durations.

OLD MAN'S BEARD
HOW TO

Supplement: Tincture of Usnea (Old Man's Beard)
1/2 teaspoon three times daily for 3-5 days.

Topical:

STEP 1 Make a tea from fresh or dried plant.

STEP 2 Chill the tea to refrigerated temperature.

STEP 3 Soak a clean cloth in the chilled tea and apply directly to the affected area of the skin for 15-20 minutes. As your body warms the area, the increased circulation allows more absorption of the herbal medicine tea.

STEP 4 Dry the area thoroughly by blotting.

STEP 5 Repeat two more times daily.

STEP 6 Use until there's no sign of fungal infection.

OLD MAN'S BEARD
CAUTIONS

Liver disease: Do not take Old Man's Beard if you have liver disease.

Mold allergy: Because it's a lichen, some people who have a true allergic reaction to mold also react to Old Man's Beard. If you're allergic to mold, test a small area of skin with tea before ingesting this herb.

5 THYME

Thyme is one of my favorite antifungal herbs because of its versatility. You can use the plant fresh or dried, as an essential oil, eaten in food, or taken in capsules. It grows like a weed and is hard for non-gardeners to kill. It's a wonderful herb to add to a kitchen or container garden because of its tenacity. It's this same tenacity that makes it a perfect match for mold.

Thyme is one of the most widely acting antifungal plants we have. It's effective against mold, but also against parasites, protozoans, and a host of other questionable characters that exist in biofilm. While Old Man's Beard goes to the sinuses, Thyme goes to the lungs. It's helpful for the mold sufferer who gets lung infections or bronchitis frequently.

Thyme's essential oil, thymol, is stimulating and drying. It improves bad breath by breaking up fungal biofilms on the teeth. You may know it better as Listerine. Essential oil of Thyme can also be inhaled for chronic sinus or lung issues.

Despite its high safety profile, I use Thyme in short durations to maximize efficacy.

THYME

HOW TO

Steam Inhalation:

STEP 1 Boil 3 tablespoons of dried Thyme in 4 quarts of water.

STEP 2 Once boiling, remove from heat.

STEP 3 Lean your head over the pot without touching it.

STEP 4 Cover your head and the pot with a dish towel.

STEP 5 Breathe deeply through your nose for 5 minutes.

Tincture of Thyme: Take 1/2 teaspoon of Thyme tincture 2-3 times per day for up to 10 days.

THYME

CAUTIONS

Taste: Many people can't tolerate Thyme as a tea, so I generally recommend using it as a tincture or in pill form.

Nausea: Because of its high safety profile, Thyme can be ingested in very large amounts. If taken in too much quantity, it can irritate the stomach and cause nausea. If you have this side effect, reduce your dose.

Pregnancy: Use Thyme cautiously while pregnant. Avoid ingesting essential oil of Thyme, or thymol, during pregnancy.

6 OIL OF OREGANO

Of all the antifungals listed, Oil of Oregano is the harshest. My patients refer to it lovingly as "the bomb". While it can be a little tough on the gut, it can help by mandating order over a disordered digestion. When bloating or irritable bowel goes haywire, Oil of Oregano helps to restore a more normal flora balance.

Oil of Oregano is antifungal and antibacterial. It kills bad actors, and normally peaceful inhabitants that have turned criminal because of biofilm influence. Oil of Oregano helps all areas of the body, even though all the press is about digestion. It's one of those that protects while it kills. It prevents oxidative damage at the cellular level, while destroying mold. It also has anticancer properties. Oil of Oregano is a true overachiever mold soldier.

Oil of Oregano is available as a concentrated extract. An extract of 10:1 is equivalent to eating a few tablespoons of oregano. The extract packs more punch than simply eating oregano in your diet.

OIL OF OREGANO
HOW TO

Food: Add oregano to cooking for an extra fungal fighting bonus.

Supplement: Take 150mg of a 10:1 extract 1-2 times daily for up to 7 days.

OIL OF OREGANO
CAUTIONS

Digestive upset: While Oil of Oregano normally helps digestion, in some people it can be too harsh and cause digestive upset. Try taking it with food to minimize this effect.

Flora imbalance: Many mold-sick people who use Oil of Oregano frequently feel best combining it with probiotics to rebalance the flora in the gut.

Prescription Antifungal Medications: Since you need a doctor to prescribe these, I won't cover them at length, other than to let you know that they exist if you and your doctor feel it's necessary. It isn't a failure to use a prescription antifungal medication. Everyone's situation is different. These can bring much needed relief and have their place.

Whole body antifungal drugs are fluconazole and nystatin. Nasal antifungal medications are amphotericin B, ketoconazole, and nystatin. Each is better for different uses, depending on whether you also have a yeast problem in conjunction with your mold sickness. This can be quite common. In practice, I tend to use these in short bursts to knock back fungal populations, especially when symptoms become barriers to sticking with the plan.

NASAL ANTIFUNGALS

With your whole-body antifungals on board, you're ready to target the colonies in your sinuses.

Do all mold-sick people need sinus treatment, even if they don't have sinus problems? Probably. If your score on the Crista Mold Questionnaire shows Possible or Probable mold sickness, I say yes. If you have urine mycotoxins, most definitely yes.

If you've been exposed to a water-damaged building, your sinus fungi have become bad actors—bad actors that need to be eradicated. If allowed to exist, biofilm mold and its friends actively poison the rest of your body with toxins, and seed other areas of your body to colonize.

I find that if you treat the body without treating the sinuses, the colonies in the sinuses keep some survivalists behind. The minute you stop treatment, the colonies send scouts and rebuild. Mold is tenacious, not something you want skulking around in hard-to-reach sinus cavities.

The best way to get antifungals up into all the crooks and crevices of your sinuses is to use a nebulizer. See the *Resources* section for nebulizer options. That said, I'm not against nasal sprays. Usually, nasal sprays work just fine IF you're doing all your orange peeling homework and taking whole-body antifungals.

To adequately eradicate mold and its bad-guy friends from your sinuses, you need tools that kill the whole gang—mold, bacteria, etc—as well as things that dissolve biofilm slime so they can't hide. I typically rotate two to three different nasal remedies at a time.

Nasal treatments include:

7 Essential oils
8 Colloidal silver
9 Ozone
10 Xylitol

7 ESSENTIAL OILS

Essential oils guard our sinus and respiratory passages. They're particularly good tools for the mold sufferer who has chronic sinus or lung problems. I recommend inhaling them rather than ingesting them. Even though many essential oils are safe to be ingested, it's best to get guidance from a trained practitioner before ingesting essential oils.

The list below includes essential oils that are effective at crippling or killing mold. They also have broad-spectrum action against bacteria. They make perfect weapons against bad-guy biofilm in the sinuses. Essential oils evaporate easily, so they can travel into the crevices of our sinuses where other medicines can't reach.

One of the problems with killing sinus mold is that it will spit out extra mycotoxins in defense, like gas bombs. But essential oils take care of this problem. Like a bomb squad, essential oils prevent and neutralize mycotoxins. So if you do have sinus biofilm, inhaling essential oils regularly reduces the impact of the mold on the rest of your body.

Choose scents that appeal to you. Use organic sources whenever possible. Essential oils are concentrates of the plant, which means if pesticides were used in growing that plant, the pesticides are concentrated too.

The following essential oils are effective at **killing sinus mold**:

Cedar leaf (Thuja plicata)
Rosemary leaf (Rosmarinus officinalis)
Ajwain seed (Trachyspermum copticum L.)
Holy Basil leaf (Ocimum sanctum, O. basilicum)
Cumin seed (Cuminum cyminum L.)
Tea tree (Maleleuca alternifolia)
Thyme leaf (Thymus vulgaris)
Cloves (Eugenia caryophyllata, E. aromatica)
Frankincense (Boswellia species)
Eucalyptus (Eucalyptus species)
Scotch Pine (Pinus sylvestris)

You can make your own blend easily at home. Follow these steps, or watch my video. Search Essential Oil Spray on DrCrista.com.

ESSENTIAL OILS

MAKE YOUR OWN BLEND

STEP 1 Use a 1-ounce glass spray bottle with a nasal diffuser. These can be found at most health food stores or online.

STEP 2 Fill the bottle 3/4 full with saline.

STEP 3 Pick two to three essential oils from the list above.

STEP 4 Drop 5 drops of each essential oil into the bottle.

STEP 5 Shake well before spraying.

STEP 6 Spritz into the air and slowly inhale the mist cloud through your nose to see if you like the smell of the blend.

STEP 7 Adjust blend by adding individual essential oils 5 drops at a time until you've created a mix that's pleasing to you.

If you aren't up for this level of involvement but want to use essential oils as part of your plan, try some of the essential oil nasal sprays on the market. I've had mixed results with different brands, and have had difficulty finding organic sources. See the *Resources* section for more information.

Dosing is an art form. There's no firm dose established in the scientific literature, so I've recommended what has worked best for my mold-sick patients. It's typical to require quite a bit initially, then less and less as you heal. Don't stop until all mycotoxins are gone plus at least one month, even if it's just once per day.

As a core part of your FIGHT tool, choose antifungal essential oils from above, and use a minimum of once per day, and a maximum of five times per day.

ESSENTIAL OILS

HOW TO

STEP 1 Point the nasal spray bottle away from your face, and pump one time to prime the unit.

STEP 2 Insert the tip as high into your nostril as possible.

STEP 3 Tip your head back, and pump 2 sprays into your nose. Sniff lightly, if needed, to retain as much of the medicine in your sinuses as possible. Try to avoid swallowing the medicine. You want it to remain in your sinuses.

STEP 4 Repeat with the other nostril.

STEP 5 To maximize the therapy, use the following steps after you've sprayed antifungals up your nose:
-lie down on your side for 30 seconds
-flip to the other side for 30 seconds
-hang your head between your knees for 30 seconds

I can't emphasize enough how much I suggest this added insurance policy. You'd be surprised how effective positioning can be. Taking a few extra minutes with each dose saves you months of continued treatment.

ESSENTIAL OILS

CAUTIONS

Nose bleeds: While using nasal antifungals, it's pretty common to get streaks of blood on facial tissue when you blow your nose. If you develop nose bleeds that don't stop easily, stop nasal treatment for a week and then resume.

Chemical sensitivity: Some mold-sick people can't tolerate essential oils. Essential oils contain aldehydes that are similar in composition to mold gases. This tends to be due to genetics. If you don't feel well around essential oils, avoid them. There are many other tools to choose from. Consider using bee propolis nasal spray. Make sure the company tests for mycotoxin contamination, as this is common.

8 COLLOIDAL SILVER

To address the characters other than mold that are living inside your sinuses, colloidal silver is used. Colloidal silver is considered a broad-spectrum antimicrobial, meaning it addresses many different kinds of bacteria. It's safe to use as a nasal spray long-term.

Use colloidal silver nasal spray once daily in conjunction with antifungal nasal treatments. Use 1 hour or more away from any other nasal treatment.

COLLOIDAL SILVER

HOW TO

STEP 1 Point the nasal spray bottle away from your face, and pump one time to prime the unit.

STEP 2 Insert the tip as high into your nostril as possible.

STEP 3 Tip your head back and pump 2 sprays into your nose. Sniff lightly, if needed, to retain as much of the medicine in your sinuses as possible. Try to avoid swallowing the medicine. You want it to remain in your sinuses.

STEP 4 Repeat with the other nostril.

STEP 5 To maximize the therapy, use the following steps after you've sprayed xylitol up your nose:
-lie down on your side for 30 seconds
-flip to the other side for 30 seconds
-hang your head between your knees for 30 seconds

I can't emphasize enough how much I suggest this added insurance policy. You'd be surprised how effective positioning can be. Taking a few extra minutes with each dose saves you months of continued treatment.

COLLOIDAL SILVER

CAUTIONS

Flora imbalance: If swallowed repeatedly, colloidal silver can cause an imbalance of the gut flora by killing off the good guys along with the bad. This may cause gas, constipation, and/or diarrhea. Try to avoid swallowing the nasal spray. Taking a daily probiotic can help rebalance flora until digestion normalizes.

Herx/Die-off reaction: Initially, colloidal silver can cause a massive die-off of bad bacteria in the sinuses. People describe feeling fluey with aches, fatigue, sore throat, and swollen lymph nodes. If this happens, temporarily stop the colloidal silver to let your body catch up.

9 OZONE

Ozone is an extremely powerful and reliable antifungal agent. It's also purported to dissolve biofilms. Even though ozone is harmful to breathe into the lungs, it can be administered in a medically targeted way inside the sinuses to clear mold and its bad-guy microbial friends. If used correctly, ozone imposes very little harm as compared to its massive results.

Ozone requires a doctor's supervision, so I won't discuss it much, other than to tell you that it exists and is a wonderful antifungal tool.

Dr. Neil Nathan, highly experienced mold-treating physician

and mold illness educator, offers details about using nasal ozone in his book, *Mold & Mycotoxins*.

10 XYLITOL

Xylitol is a biofilm buster, meaning that it breaks up the slime layer protecting mold and its co-conspirators. Remember, once you're exposed to a water-damaged building, the bad dudes that thrived in that sick building have moved into your sinuses. They survive in a biofilm, and it's literally a film of slime mixed with bad-guy microbes. While antifungals work on bad-guy mold, and colloidal silver works on bad-guy bacteria, xylitol chips away at the slime they're hiding in.

Don't add this to your regimen too soon. Wait until you feel like you've gotten a leg up before starting xylitol to make sure your body can handle what's uncovered.

Xylitol is a very palatable remedy to spray up your nose. It's soothing to sinuses and tastes sweet if swallowed.

I recommend using xylitol nasal spray once daily in conjunction with antifungal nasal treatments. Use 1 hour or more away from any other nasal treatment.

XYLITOL

HOW TO

STEP 1 Point the nasal spray bottle away from your face, and pump one time to prime the unit.

STEP 2 Insert the tip as high into your nostril as possible.

STEP 3 Tip your head back and pump 2 sprays into your nose. Sniff lightly, if needed, to retain as much of the medicine in your sinuses as possible. Try to avoid swallowing the medicine. You want it to remain in your sinuses.

STEP 4 Repeat with the other nostril.

STEP 5 To maximize the therapy, use the following steps after you've sprayed xylitol up your nose:
-lie down on your side for 30 seconds
-flip to the other side for 30 seconds
-hang your head between your knees for 30 seconds

I can't emphasize enough how much I suggest this added insurance policy. You'd be surprised how effective positioning can be. Taking a few extra minutes with each dose saves you months of continued treatment.

XYLITOL

CAUTIONS

Herx/Die-off reaction: If used too early, xylitol can reveal more mold than your body is ready to handle, and you can get sicker. Add biofilm busting after symptoms have reduced to a tolerable level, and only as long as whole-body antifungals are on board.

Prescription Nasal Antifungals: Prescription nasal antifungals may need to be added if other methods aren't working. Monitor your urine mycotoxin tests and discuss this with your doctor.

Alternate Nostril Breathing: If you have significant sinus symptoms, consider learning Alternate Nostril Breathing, a yoga technique that is especially powerful immediately after using the nasal treatment.

Spray Mists: Some of my patients spritz essential oils on and around themselves to reduce symptoms. They may spritz hourly to reduce sinus and lung complications. Others only need a spritz before bed so they can breathe when lying down. Experiment to find what works for you.

Zum Mist is a current favorite. They have exquisite blends using many of the essential oils mentioned above, however, they don't come in nasal spray form. Do not spray these up your nose.

FINISH THE JOB

The following additional support tools don't necessarily kill mold, but are necessary to completely heal from mold.

Finish the job involves:

11 Biofilm Busters *expose hidden mold*
12 Herx Helpers *help you stay on target*
13 Reintroduction *get your life back to normal*

11 BIOFILM BUSTERS

Biofilms are a problem in mold sickness. The bad guys that thrive in water-damaged buildings move into your body and transform your natural flora into a slime of bad actors. When I think of biofilms, I think of the movie Mad Max; everyone in it for himself, competing, and creating a toxic wasteland.

I've talked about biofilm as an issue of the sinuses and gut. But if you have mold sickness, biofilms have the potential to form in many places around your body. The sinuses and gut are just the urban hubs for bad-guy biofilms. Biofilms can happen on your teeth, in your root canals, on joint replacements, on your contact lenses, and so on. If you're sick from mold, any biofilm location can host survivors.

It's a good idea to decimate these hideouts…IF you're up to it.

One mistake I see with mold treatment is that people start biofilm busters too early in their treatment plan. Breaking up biofilm will cause two reactions. First, the bad guys scatter and search for other places to hide, which can cause a flare up of mold symptoms. Second, it causes the bad guys to wage war against whichever tissue is hosting a hideout. Wait until you have things in place to handle these reactions.

Timing is everything.

How do you know when it's time for biofilm busting? It's time to add biofilm busters when you've hit a plateau, or if you can't stop treatment without getting sicker. Otherwise, hold off. Don't add these until you're successfully taking whole-body antifungals and targeted nasal antifungals and feeling okay.

There can be an art to biofilm busting. Leftover biofilm can keep mold-sick people from getting better, even if they've done everything right. I've learned the most from Dr. Paul Anderson—about this and many other intricacies of mold fighting. If you and your doctor have determined that stubborn biofilm is an issue for you, your doctor can get specific training with Dr. Anderson at his website (consultdranderson.com).

Most agents that bust biofilm are called enzymes. Enzymes digest stuff. They literally digest the slime. Enzymes are most potent if taken away from meals. Otherwise, they just help you digest what you ate rather than the slime.

BIOFILM BUSTERS
HOW TO

Enzymes: Many foods are naturally high in enzymes. Fresh, raw pineapple and papaya are examples. I haven't found food sources to be strong enough to get at biofilm without causing sores in the mouth or on the tongue, so this is one I supplement.

Supplement: Take a multi-enzyme supplement, 1 capsule 1-2 times daily, away from meals by 1 hour.

BIOFILM BUSTERS
CAUTIONS

Herx/Die-off reaction: Stop taking enzymes if you have a herxheimer reaction. Use the Herx tools in the next section, and try again at a later time, after you've killed more mold.

Digestive irritation: In some, enzymes can further irritate an already irritated digestive lining. This causes heartburn and sometimes symptoms of an ulcer. If this occurs, try taking the enzyme with meals. If it's still causing irritation, stop taking enzymes.

12 HERX HELPERS

Here's a list of things to try if you feel worse while working to get better. A Herxheimer reaction occurs when you kill more mold than your body can handle.

- **Adjust treatment:** Many times people need to reduce, pause, suspend, cut doses, or make some adjustment to their treatment plan in order to move through a Herx die-off reaction.
- **Epsom salt bath:** Use 2 cups Epsom salts in one bath. Soak for 20-30 minutes. This is safe to use daily.
- **Lemon juice:** Drink the juice of 2 lemons in 8 ounces of spring water. Repeat as needed.
- **Alka-Seltzer Gold:** Use one tablet in 8 ounces of spring water. This can be alternated with lemon juice.
- **Bieler's Broth fast:** See the description below.

HERX HELPERS
HOW TO

Bieler's Broth: Eat nothing but this soup for a minimum of 2 days. Eat as much as desired. Then add a protein of choice for another 2 days. If you're feeling improvement, slowly add back your normal dietary items.

RECIPE

BIELER'S BROTH

Ingredients (use only organic ingredients)

4 cups spring water
3 medium zucchini, coarsely chopped
4 stalks celery, coarsely chopped
1 pound string beans, tipped
1 bunch parsley, stems removed

THE END OF DR. BIELER'S INGREDIENTS

Optional additions for mold recovery:

Up to ¼ cup each of nettles, beet greens, or dandelion leaves.
(NOTE: Handle raw nettles with gloves to prevent stinging. Once cooked, they no longer sting.)
1-2 cloves garlic or 1/4 cup chopped onions, or both (optional)
1/4 cup olive oil or butter (optional)

* * * * * * * * * * * * * * *

In a large pot, sauté celery, zucchini, string beans, garlic, and onions in oil or butter for 5-7 minutes.

Add water, nettles, beet greens, and **dandelion greens**, and bring to a boil.

Boil for about 10 minutes or until all vegetables are bright green and tender.

Remove from heat and **add parsley**.

Use an immersion blender or food processor to blend until smooth.

Spice to taste using salt, pepper, or other desired spices.

Quoting Dr. Jillian Stansbury, **"use spices with wild abandon."**

Another version of this recipe can be found in Nourishing Traditions by Sally Fallon.

13 REINTRODUCTION

If you've had to give up favorite foods, beverages, or hobbies because of this blasted mold thing, there's hope. Most things on the list of avoidances can be brought back after you've completed treatment.

Tips for REINTRODUCTION...

- Bring back only one thing at a time
- Wait for 4 days to see how you feel
- If you have a bad reaction IN ANY WAY, remove the AVOIDANCE item again
- If you've had a bad reaction, you may need to restart mold killers for a short time to reconquer the mold

Remember, mold is tenacious and an opportunist. I've had many patients that thought they were out of the woods be taken down by circumstances or holidays. Only a few days of overeating sweets contributes to fungal overload and the return of mold symptoms. Return to the plan that got you better. Rely on it until you feel yourself again, and then wean slowly. It usually only takes a few weeks if you listen to your body and act nimbly.

ENOUGH ALREADY!

Fighting mold can sort of feel like fighting zombies. Just when you think you've killed it all the way dead, it can surface again. You hit it with daily antifungal tea, pulse stronger whole-body antifungals, and spray essential oils up your nose. And the day after you stop any one of those things, one of your symptoms returns, and you think, "you've gotta be kidding me!"

Nope.

Not kidding.

Stay on your treatments longer than you think you need to. Mold will come back like a zombie. Just because your symptoms have become tolerable and you have a good score on the Crista Mold Questionnaire, does not mean you're in the clear. I'm sorry, but it's true. Stay on your stuff until ALL mold symptoms are gone, plus one more month. I don't want you to have to read this book over again. Once was plenty.

I know from experience that you can get better. Work the plan, one step at a time. Keep moving forward.

Moss can't grow on a rolling stone…

…or in a healthy building.

PART 3
BUILDINGS

Indoor Mold is Bad

Period.

There's no such thing as "safe" or "not the bad kind" of mold or mildew existing inside a building. Any fungus of any kind growing inside a building is bad news.

You may have gotten sick from a current or a past environment, a fact that surprises many people. Remember, it invades your body and your belongings, so you can bring an old problem with you wherever you go.

Take a long, hard look at environments where you've spent significant amounts of time. Do a thorough historical assessment to include all environments. Include places where you lived, worked, prayed, exercised, volunteered, and vacationed. Consider times when you may have been more susceptible, for example when you were extra stressed or not getting enough sleep. Mold will capitalize on those moments.

STORY | **CARPET MUSHROOMS**

When I was in college, a friend called with a strange invitation. She asked if I wanted to come see her carpet mushrooms. Of course I said yes. Who could pass that up? They were as funny looking as they sound. There were literally three species of mushroom crops sprouting up through her carpet. If there were smartphones back then, I would've snapped a pic and shared it with an LOL caption.

My friend rented the small cottage while it was winter. It was an adorable repurposed barn. As things thawed that spring though, it became clear that there were some problems with the remodel. We didn't know about the dangers of mold. Instead, we laughed about it. It became a funny story to tell at parties.

In the weeks that followed the carpet mushroom episode, she began to develop health problems. It started as acne and fatigue, then nausea and decreased appetite, then cyclical vomiting syndrome. Within the next three months, she developed kidney disease.

She became too sick to go to school or work. She didn't have family near, so she came to stay with me after an episode of cyclical vomiting that didn't seem like it would ever stop. I was so worried about her. Her doctors were too. There didn't seem to be any explanation for why this previously fit and healthy 20-year-old woman was falling apart so quickly.

After a few weeks out of the cottage, she started to feel a little better. At an appointment, her observant chiropractor asked about her living environment. When we joked about the carpet mushrooms, he looked horrified. He educated us that her cottage was the problem. It was literally killing her.

After he made the connection, we both felt kind of dumb. How hadn't either of us made that connection? Of course it was a problem having mushrooms grow through the carpet; much more than a building problem, it was also a health problem. I think we were both too busy managing the latest health crisis to step back and think holistically. ✺

3.1
Building Diagnosis

Test with the experts. If there is any water intrusion in your home, get a certified mold inspector to test for mold. Well-trained mold inspectors are like doctors for buildings. They can diagnose a building's issues by knowing where to test, which test to use, and what material to sample. My personal go-to person, Martine Davis, is a certified building biologist, and is brilliant. I've listed my recommendations for inspectors in other areas of the country in the *Resources* section. Many also offer long-distance consultation services as well.

Check credentials. They matter. A lot of untrained people are out there taking advantage of homeowners in crisis mode. Take time to do it right. Search for people with one or more of these credentials.

MOLD INSPECTORS
CREDENTIALS TO LOOK FOR

- **BBEC** (Building Biology Environmental Consultant)
- **ACAC** (American Council for Accredited Certification)
- **IICRC** (Institute of Inspection, Cleaning, and Restoration Certification)

That's how you find the ones who really know their stuff. They test your house for mold spores, spore fragments, and evidence of mycotoxins. If you test without their guidance, you have a higher chance of not finding the mold, even if it's there. You also may lose out on insurance coverage for your remediation because you didn't have a certified test.

LET REMEDIATORS REMEDIATE AND TESTERS TEST

Don't let the remediation company replace the independent certified mold inspector. That's a major conflict of interest. If there is a mold problem that needs remediation, you absolutely should test after the remediation is complete to make sure the mold is gone. The only post-remediation test you should trust is the independent certified mold inspector's test. Remediation companies certainly test after they clean up, but that's for their own quality controls. You need an independent advocate.

It's estimated that 1 in 3 remediations have had to either be redone, or the families had to call the remediators back to take more materials out. Usually it's discovered the hard way, by getting sicker. That's a lot of expense, hassle, mess, and lost health that didn't need to happen. The certified inspector can work with you and your remediation company to ensure a thorough remediation the first time. In the *Remediation* section, I've listed some simple tips to follow.

I have yet to find a remediation company that addresses mycotoxins. If someone is still sick after a thorough remediation, it's likely because the mycotoxins haven't been remediated. I've guided my patients on mycotoxin remediation and have verified the methods by post-testing the materials. But none of the methods have gone through scientific rigor to make sure the results are repeatable. Keep a lookout for developments in this field.

HOME MOLD TEST MYTH

When it comes to testing your home, I really want to discourage DIY testing. Tests from a big-box store fail miserably because 90% of the toxic indoor molds don't grow on that culture medium. So, you're only catching 10% of the indoor molds. That's not a good test.

If you've already used one of these, and it found mold, trust it. Your affected area is apparently exposed to enough indoor air that it could be picked up. Not necessarily a good thing for the health of the inhabitants, but good that it was discovered.

If a DIY test has come back clean, ignore it. The only thing it's giving you is a false sense of security. People then go looking around for other causes thinking they've ruled out mold, while mold is happily expanding its territory in their homes. Independent certified mold inspectors are worth the money. I've seen too many times that families scrimp on that decision, but then spend way more money chasing mystery health conditions.

The other issue with testing the most toxic molds is that they're sticky and gooey. They don't easily float around. They're also usually trapped behind building materials, which means there aren't aerated spores to be caught by air sampling. Inspectors often have to go digging to find these.

But take caution before disrupting that moldy area.

DON'T POKE THE BEAR

Don't disrupt any suspicious area without taking precautions. Don't decide, "Oh, well, it looks bad, we can see it's mold, whatever, we'll just take it out." When you do that, you release broken spore fragments and mycotoxins into your air and into your lungs.

Spore fragments can lodge deep into the lung tissue causing long-term respiratory problems. All mycotoxins seep through lungs, which your body then has to detoxify. In addition, mycotoxins are supremely absorbable through the skin. You can make yourself very sick.

Who You Gonna Call? **Mold Busters!**

How You Gonna Find Them? **Mold Testers!**

Ask your certified inspector for recommendations on good remediation companies in your area. They know who's doing good work. It's normal to hire your inspector to oversee your remediation project. This works as a really nice partnership with all sides working together to make sure you come back to a healthy house.

MYCOTOXIN DUST TEST

Sometimes you don't have a certified mold inspector nearby. Not to worry, many inspectors will do long-distance consultations. One test they often ask you to help with is the mycotoxin dust test, because it can be collected by you in your own space. The inspector can provide you with a kit.

The mycotoxin dust test is a handy way to check whether a building is having, or has had, a mold problem. It only tells you whether mycotoxins are present in the building environment. The test does not, however, tell where the problem is, how long it has been a problem, or even if it's a current issue. That's where the experts come in.

My reason for telling you about this is to make sure you're collecting the best sample possible. Technique is everything. Collect dust samples from multiple places around the house, and areas where dust has been allowed to accumulate for many months.

COLLECT from the top surfaces of... picture frames
tall shelves
books
kitchen cabinets
trim around closets

Avoid testing around windows and doors to the outside, as these may be contaminated with outdoor molds that came in with the breeze. These areas don't reflect the health of an indoor environment.

3.2
Remediation

A "PRECAUTION"-ARY TALE

You must take precautions to stay well during remediation. What precautions? The most valuable precaution is AVOIDANCE. Stay out of buildings, vehicles, RVs, etc that have had water-damage that hasn't been properly addressed. There's no amount of air filtration, open windows, or fans that can keep up with mold's stealth ability to make boatloads of toxins.

A 1-inch square of toxic mold contains one million spores. Each day, that many spores can create enough gases and toxins to fill multiple balloons. If you decide you're going to skip remediation and filter the air, it won't work. You're out numbered, and you'll eventually get sick.

CONTAINMENT

Containment is another important precaution. Containment means sealing off the sick area with plastic. When you disturb mold, it has a poisonous survival reaction. It spits out more mycotoxins than normal and shoots baby spores into the air for survival of the species. When mold breaks apart, its toxic mold guts spill other chemicals into the environment.

Containment includes the use of negative air. Air is sucked outside from the sealed off area so that if anything goes "poof" it goes outside instead of into your home. This is a key reason to trust professionals to do the cleanup. They have all the tools and the training.

Sometimes, containment is even necessary when testing an area, if the sampling requires a fair amount of disruption to building materials. In our house, enough mold toxin got out through the drill hole in our ceiling to make us sick. Now, fair enough. I am a mold canary. But if a teeny drill hole can release enough toxicity to make a mold canary sick, how much does it take to make a non-canary sick? Tearing out carpet? Knocking out some drywall? Is it really worth getting sick to find out? Seal test areas with plastic. Contain it before it gets out of hand.

PROTECTIVE GEAR

If you must go into a water-damaged environment to assess damage to your property, I recommend wearing the proper protective gear. I've done quite a few phone consults with doctors treating patients who made themselves sick by going into their water-damaged homes after a hurricane or flood. The sickest were the people who did their own clean-up without protective gear. The problem is they didn't fully understand the dangers of mold. They went in without any personal protective gear, not even gloves, and poisoned themselves.

Proper protective gear to block spore inhalation is important, but don't forget the gases. Active and dying molds secrete mycotoxins, as well as gases such as aldehydes and alcohols.

These gases are infinitesimally small. They can seep through all mask filters and clothing. And they don't necessarily have a scent. This is why I don't recommend DIY remediation.

DORKS STAY HEALTHY

Don't be afraid to look like a total dork when you show up in your mold-protective getup. Remediators wear it too. That's how they stay well despite working amongst toxic mold all day. They get it.

Everything needs to be covered head to toe with the least amount of exposed areas. Here's a list of things you need on your body before you go into a potentially sick environment.

LIST OF THINGS you Need...

- disposable Tyvek suit with hood (toss after each exposure)
- safety glasses (clean with bleach after each use)
- silicone respirator with disposable filters
- P100 respirator filters (toss after each exposure)
- double gloves (toss after each exposure)
- shoe booties (toss after each exposure)

When you step out of the environment, peel off the gloves, suit and booties, and throw them away. Change the filters on your mask. Clean your mask and safety glasses with bleach or essential oils.

Don't just jump in your car and infect your car with the same problem. When you get to your safe house, head directly to the shower to make sure mycotoxins are rinsed off your skin rather than absorbed.

WHO STAYS OUT

As I said in the beginning, mycotoxins are harmful to all living beings: people, animals, and plants. Some get affected quicker and harder than others. It's simply a matter of how much, for how long, and genetic sensitivity. Some people have a hard time getting rid of the toxins, while others can metabolize them efficiently.

Currently there are no respirator mask filters that filter down to the mycotoxin size. There are some room-size air filters that can, but not respirator mask filters. That size of a mask filter would restrict breathing. So until technology catches up with mold, the following people should never go into a water-damaged building—not even for a second, not even to assess the damage, not even to meet with insurance, and not even with a mask on. Just stay out.

People who need to STAY OUT...

pregnant women
women who are nursing
young children
people with respiratory conditions
people with liver disease
people with kidney disease
people with immune deficiency
people with cancer
genetically mold sensitive (canaries)

PROTECTIVE PLANT PUSHER

The remediators who worked on my house will tell you that I'm a milk thistle pusher. Because I know the harmful effects of mold, I wanted to make sure they were protecting their bodies from exposure to mycotoxins that pass through mask filters. The research tells us that a minimum daily dose of 750mg is required to achieve milk thistle's protective benefits. I think all remediators should be doing this. My only caution is that if they're taking a medication that is processed through the cytochrome p450 system, they need to see a mold-literate doctor for dose adjustment.

DR. J'S REMEDIATION TIPS

I'm a scientist at heart, but I treat bodies, not buildings. For buildings, I turn to my friend and compadre, mold expert and certified building biologist Martine Davis. Martine has taught me a lot about moldy buildings. Combining that knowledge with my exquisite sensitivity to mold makes me the perfect anti-mold advocate—and a royal pain for any remediation crew that has to work with me, I'm sure.

As I helped patients through their remediations, I did home visits and got to take part in scientifically testing materials that both my patients and I reacted to. I learned about testing and watched remediation techniques. Throughout the years, I developed some rules of thumb to guide remediation, protect my patients, and reduce "do-overs".

REMEDIATION rules of thumb...

1. No spray and pray
2. No seal and deal
3. When in doubt, cut it out
4. Take out more than you think

1 NO SPRAY & PRAY

The sprays used by most remediators are stain removers. They commonly don't contain enough antifungal chemical activity to account for the amount of moisture they add to the water-damaged material.

These sprays effectively water the mold, and can welcome other species to jump into the mix. I learned this because I tested it. Read below or visit my video-blog page on DrCrista.com.

STORY | **NO SPRAY AND PRAY**

Throughout the remediation in my own home, I had the perfect opportunity to run mini controlled studies. I could test the same materials from the same house that had been under the same circumstances of water-damage and exposure to mold for the same amount of time. The only difference was whether a material had been remediated or not. Rather than conducting these studies in a sterile lab, I got to see what happens post-remediation in a house that once hosted biofilm.

Here's how I came up with the phrase "no spray and pray". One section of my basement was moldy and needed remediation. All building materials from that area were removed from floor to ceiling, including drywall, insulation, and the bottom 4 inches of some studs. The sill plate (the 2x4 board that runs horizontally along the basement floor to which studs are nailed) was left in place.

The sill plate was remediated according to current quality standards of remediation, which involved wire brush scrubbing, HEPA vacuuming, and being treated with a commercial mold-killing spray. Because I was using a remediation company recommended by my certified mold inspector, I knew I was getting top-shelf remediation.

I started to become concerned about the sill plate. If the lower part of the studs attached to the sill plate needed to be removed, then wouldn't the sill plate be bad as well? And how sure were we that the mold-killing spray did the job?

The top of the sill plate looked okay. Only half of this particular sill plate board was exposed and treated, because the other half was left beneath the normal, not mold-affected wall. To be sure, I asked for the space under the exposed sill plate to be tested.

The test came back that the sill plate had Stachybotrys chartarum (toxic black mold) wedged between the bottom of the sill plate board and the cement floor. So now it needed to be removed to achieve a complete remediation of the area, which was possible since it wasn't part of the structural support of the building.

The remediators were so overbooked, they couldn't get me back on their schedule for another three weeks. When they returned, they removed the entire sill plate, including the adjacent wall that sat above it. We had the entire board now to run some tests. They took photos and samples of the "clean" non-remediated section of the board, the remediated section, and the junction between the two sections.

Results were stunning. The remediation reduced the quantity of spores overall, but some survivors were still present. And here's the scariest part. The treated side of the board, the area sprayed with the mold-killing spray, not only had the same mold as the untreated side, but now had two additional species that weren't there three weeks prior. These were more toxic microbes that had never been there before.

It's as if the mold-killing spray watered the biofilm and encouraged new bad-guy characters to move in. The analogy I thought of was what happens in unruly societies; when enough small-time petty-crime criminals get knocked out of the way, organized crime comes in and takes over.

This is how I come to the conclusion that if at all possible, and as long as it's not structurally required, remove any and all sick building material. ✺

Ok, so if mold-killing sprays add more bad guys, what do you do if you can't remove it? What if the sick area is structurally critical? I wish I had a scientifically-based answer for you. Most of the studies done on the commercially available sprays are not done within a sick building. I think this is a short-coming, but one that almost can't be helped. Every sick building grows its own unique brand of biofilm, its own mix of microbes and microbial toxins. Therefore, products would need to be tested in about 100 different sick buildings, and then repeated within the exact same conditions. That's not realistic. We simply don't have the breadth and rigor of scientific studies to have a tidy solution for this.

In our home, there were a few structural members that couldn't be removed. We had to get creative without affecting the structural integrity of the home. I consulted with a builder. The options were to hand plane or sand an ultra-thin layer off the member to remove the surface colonies. This is where the largest population would live to get access to moisture and oxygen. I had concerns about choosing the option to use a sander because it would create excessive amounts of fragments and mycotoxins. Remember, these are so small, they can get through a mask filter. We decided on a combination of the two.

After the top layer was removed, the remediators wire brush scrubbed and HEPA vacuumed multiple times. Then they allowed me to use essential oils and peroxide to treat the members. Once it tested clean, as a final step, they sealed it. Of course all this was done under containment and using the proper personal protective gear.

I was overjoyed at the results. I had absolutely no reaction to these spaces. I felt confident that the rebuild could now begin.

2 NO SEAL & DEAL

Painting over mold without treating the area isn't effective remediation. Mycotoxins and other toxic mold gases can seep through the sealant paint. It looks nicer, but it didn't take care of the problem.

3 WHEN IN DOUBT, CUT IT OUT

After working with many patients through their remediations, I learned this rule of thumb. There were less "do-over" remediations in buildings where the owner wanted the sick building material to be removed rather than treated and sealed. I know this was true in my home as well.

Most building-owners pressure remediators to leave as much material as possible. It's a natural inclination—to save money and reduce disruption to daily life—but it doesn't work. Also know that your insurance company is likely putting the same pressures on remediators to save money.

I promise you, being sick is much more expensive.

If a material can be removed, do so...even if it's hard work, and even if it costs more. Do it once thoroughly, rather than multiple times incompletely. Mold is tenacious. Retained sick building materials are perfect starter farms for new mold growth.

STORY | **CEMENT BOARD CAN'T GROW MOLD—OR CAN IT?**

I told this story at the beginning of the book about the mold in my home. Here it is in more detail or in case you missed it.

Water from the second-floor bathroom leak made it all the way to the basement by way of my kitchen on the first floor. Unseen, the water had fully saturated areas of the kitchen beneath the surface, before dripping into the basement. This involved drywall, insulation, kitchen cabinetry, and subfloor under the ceramic tile.

I never felt well in my kitchen. The signs were subtle. I felt spacey, had low energy, and would find myself lingering there not remembering what I was doing. I could only identify this after the area was remediated. I didn't notice it at the time.

Once everything was removed and remediated, I felt better—but not all the way better. I suspiciously was still reacting whenever I entered my kitchen. I couldn't help but worry. This was where our food was made, and I was definitely reacting to something. Whatever it is could be contaminating the food we eat and the plates we eat from; destroying the linings of our intestines, wrecking our immune systems, among many other problems. My concern level rose.

Like an environmentally-sensitive canary, I worried that I was nuts. Nobody else in my family seemed to have a problem. Only me, and especially my lungs. After some internal struggle, and a healthy dose of procrastination, I made a decision. I had to follow my own advice and trust myself.

At my own expense, and not validated by the scientific testing, I requested that a perimeter of tile and subfloor surrounding the water-damaged area be removed, the area where I felt the worst. This involved the incredibly arduous work of busting up the tile and cement board. God bless those remediators.

Samples of subfloor and cement board were submitted for testing, even though I was informed that cement board couldn't grow mold.

Interestingly, the cement board, which is not supposed to be able to grow mold, was hosting two species of toxic outdoor mold. These molds cause respiratory sicknesses and immune problems. People who live in desert climates are familiar with these guys because they cause something called Valley fever or desert lung, known to doctors as Coccidioidomycosis.

Apparently, the arid indoor microclimate created by cement board, if given exposure to biofilm and just enough constant moisture, will host toxic outdoor mold. It's crazy to think that a lady in Wisconsin could be infected by desert mold from Arizona from her own kitchen.

Neither the inspector nor the remediators had ever heard of such a thing. But as both admitted, they weren't sure that anyone had ever bothered to test. After the area was remediated, I had no problem being in my kitchen. ✺

4 TAKE OUT MORE THAN YOU THINK

Just like skin cancer, if you don't have clear margins, mold will grow back. A good rule of thumb is to remove 2 feet of material beyond the visibly affected area. Mold spores are microscopic. You can't see them. Spores can infect surrounding material without visual detection.

Ask your certified mold inspector to test the "clean" border material to make sure there's no mold. If there is, keep cutting. Don't rebuild until you have the assurance of clean margins. Living in studs never hurt anyone, but mold has and will.

Remediators have a hard job. It's hot underneath all that protective gear. Have compassion as you're asking for this extra measure and expect to pay a little more. Maybe even buy them lunch.

You can either pay for a thorough remediation or doctor bills. It's your choice.

3.3

Prevention

I have a little secret to tell you.

I know mold's WEAKNESSES... dryness
sunlight
air movement
dust-free spaces
lack of clutter
mold-killing essential oils

Native Americans had it figured out. Those that lived in damp environments prevented mold growth indoors by lining their wood houses with the inner bark of certain trees, like cedar. These trees are rich in essential oils that prevent mold growth. In contrast, in modern building, we are asking for mold problems. We line our houses with paper, mold's favorite food.

THE CARE AND FEEDING OF MOLD

Of course, not all water events create mold. Unfortunately though, construction methods used over the past 50 years have created the perfect storm of mold-promoting conditions. We build extremely airtight homes that both trap humidity inside, and are made of already partially digested food sources. We also seal up water pipes behind walls so there's no way to check to see if the water is staying inside them. I've learned that it's not a matter of IF water will find a way out of a pipe, it's a matter of WHEN.

The way we build homes essentially feeds and waters mold. It's as if we followed a farm manual called "The Care and Feeding of Mold"—and did exactly what mold needed to thrive in our indoor environments. It doesn't take much. Mold is a survivor species. All it needs is some food and a little bit of humidity.

HUMIDITY CONTROL VERSUS COST SAVINGS

Many people think dehumidifiers are a waste of money and an unnecessary drain on the electric bill. I can promise you that mold remediation is much more expensive.

You don't need visible water or a flood event to grow mold. You just need moisture. You may have a moldy house because your indoor environment is just too dang humid. If you also have a dusty humid environment, congratulations. You're a successful mold farmer.

Let's try to prevent that.

Get a jump on activities that increase indoor humidity. Cooking pasta? Turn the vent on. Taking a shower? Turn the vent on. High outdoor humidity? Close up and turn on the A/C, and use a dehumidifier. All basements need dehumidifiers.

Prevent future problems by managing your indoor humidity. And don't ignore water intrusions. I see a lot of wishful thinking and comments from patients like, "we thought it was no big deal," as they're talking to me from hotel rooms while their homes were being remediated. As mold expert Dr. Sandeep

Gupta teaches in his online mold course, Mold Illness Made Simple, whatever you aren't addressing will eventually address you. You're better off living in a house with exposed studs than a sick house whose mold problem is glossed over.

STORY | **ENDOTOXINS**

During the remediation of our basement, the remediators uncovered a sill plate that looked really bad. The entire outer surface looked vegetative, the way mold looks when it grows on bread. It was clear it had to go, but they asked if I wanted samples for testing first. I said "of course!"

To all of our amazement, the tests revealed very little mold—less than what is normally found in a finished basement. I called the certified building inspector and asked about this strange test result, because none of us could believe it. She recommended testing for bacterial endotoxins.

Sure enough, the bacterial endotoxins were sky high. What we assumed was a colony of mold was actually a colony of bacteria. In this case, the conditions in that specific area of the basement hosted a biofilm that was more friendly to bacteria than mold. Either way, the toxins from both are harmful and were making us sick. That board had to go! ✹

NO FINISHED BASEMENTS

I'm overall not a fan of finished basements. The building inspector I work with says she finds mold in almost every finished basement, despite the use of dehumidifiers. Basements need to breathe.

If you need the extra space for a workout area or kid play area, I'd advise putting down foam pads in small areas if you need a soft surface. When the activity is finished, lift the pads off the floor so it can breathe.

For storage, keep everything off the floor. I'm personally a fan of metal shelving that rolls, so you can load it up and roll it around every so often, so areas of foundation can breathe. Also, mold doesn't grow on the metal shelving.

Definitely keep cardboard out of basements, especially off the basement floor. All basements are too damp for cardboard. Yes, all of them…even yours.

DUST WITH GUSTO

Simply put, dust grows mold. So, dust with gusto.

This is made easier by clearing clutter and storing knick-knacks behind glass or inside curio cabinets where you can still appreciate them but aren't harmed by them. There's a correlation between mold sickness and hoarding. I'm quite sure this partially has to do with the dust levels on all the stuff.

TAKE A LOAD OFF YOUR LUNGS

You decide, which do you prefer to clean your air? Your air filter? Or your lungs? Here's a hint…one you can change, the other you can't.

That's right, be vigilant about changing your home air filters to protect your lungs from having to be the filter. I recommend changing furnace filters a minimum of 2 times per year, depending on pets, kids, and dust levels. If you have more of these, you should change it more often. For stand-alone air filtration systems, err on the early side of their recommended time frame.

Car cabin filters can host mold. I recommend changing your car cabin filter at least yearly. Time the filter replacement for the beginning of your air conditioning season.

WHAT THE 3 LITTLE PIGS CAN TEACH US

Do not build your house with sticks; instead, build your house with bricks.

YOU'RE DONE!

You know it all now. Congratulate yourself for listening to your body and taking charge of your health. Now you're armed to protect yourself from mold.

You CAN get better. Never, ever, ever lose hope. Get outside, take a breath, open the book to the first tool, AVOIDANCE, and do one small, bite-sized thing on the list. If that's even too much, ask for help. If you've tried everything in the book and still feel cruddy, look for a mold-literate doctor.

Remember, sun is mold's kryptonite.

Stay in the light.

Best of luck to you as you BREAK THE MOLD!

Resources

Keep an eye out for more video blogs on my website:
DRCRISTA.COM

Or on Facebook **@DRJILLCRISTA**

If you prefer YouTube, find my video channel by searching **#GOTMOLD, #BREAKTHEMOLD** and subscribe.

For a printable copy of the Crista Mold Questionnaire, send an email request to support@drcrista.com.

WEBSITES & SUPPORT

Environmental Working Group (ewg.org)

Dr. Ritchie Shoemaker (survivingmold.com)

Paradigm Change
(paradigmchange.me, Mold Avoiders Facebook group)

Dr. Wayne Anderson
(gordonmedical.com / team / wayne-anderson-n-d)

Dr. Paul Anderson (consultdranderson.com)

Horowitz Lyme/Multiple Systemic Infectious Disease Syndrome (MSIDS) Questionnaire
(cangetbetter.com / symptom-list)

Dr. Jill Carnahan—Low Mold Diet
(jillcarnahan.com / 2015 / 02 / 08 / low-mold-diet /)

ARTICLES & BOOKS

Clean, Green & Lean book, Dr. Walter Crinnion
(crinnionopinion.com)

Mold Warriors and Surviving Mold books and training, Dr. Ritchie Shoemaker (survivingmold.com)

Molds & Mycotoxins book, Dr. Neil Nathan
(neilnathanmd.com / books)

Why Can't I Get Better? Solving The Mystery Of Lyme & Chronic Disease book, Dr. Richard Horowitz
(cangetbetter.com)

Reversal of Cognitive Decline article, Dr. Dale Bredesen

Dirty Genes book, Dr. Benjamin Lynch (go.dirtygenes.com/books)

The Yeast Connection book, Dr. William G. Krook

Eat Right 4 Your Type book, Dr. Peter D'Adamo (dadamo.com)

Your Guide to Forest Bathing: Experience The Healing Power of Nature book, M. Amos Clifford

Nourishing Traditions (Bieler's broth recipe) book, Sally Fallon & Mary Enig

TRAINING

Environmental Health Symposium (environmentalhealthsymposium.com)

The Forum for Integrative Medicine (forumforintegrativemedicine.org)

Mold Illness Made Simple online course, Dr. Sandeep Gupta (moldillnessmadesimple.com)

Dr. Paul Anderson (consultdranderson.com)

Klinghardt Academy training, Dr. Dietrich Klinghardt (klinghardtacademy.com/Seminars-Workshops/)

Study with Tieraona training, Dr. Tieraona Lowdog (drlowdog.com/study-with-tieraona/)

Bredesen Protocol training, Dr. Dale Bredesen (drbredesen.com/thebredesenprotocol)

AANP—American Association of Naturopathic Physicians (naturopathic.org)

AIHM—Academy of Integrative Health & Medicine (aihm.org)

SIBO information & courses, Dr. Allison Siebecker
(siboinfo.com)
(sibosos.com/home-resources-2)
(thesibodoctor.com)

TESTING A BODY (requires a doctor's order)

Urine Mycotoxins: Great Plains Laboratory (greatplainslaboratory.com)

Urine Mycotoxins: RealTime Labs (realtimelab.com)

Glutathione, Health Diagnostics & Research Institute (hdri-usa.com)

Organic Acids Test Great Plains Laboratory (greatplainslabortory.com)

TESTING A BUILDING CERTIFIED INSPECTORS

MIDWEST

Indoor Environmental, Martine Davis, (airinspector.com)

NY, NJ, CT, PA, FL

Certified Mold Inspections, Inc.,
Steven Levy, CMC, CIEC, CMR, CIT, LEED AP
Cory Levy, CMI, ACAC, IICRC
(findingthemold.com)

SOUTHERN CALIFORNIA

The Mold Guy, Mark Levy, CMC, CIEC, CMR, CIT, LEED AP (themoldguyinc.com)

We Inspect, Brian Karr (yesweinspect.com)

TESTING A BUILDING MYCOTOXINS

Real Time Labs (realtimelab.com)

FIND A DOCTOR

Go see a Naturopathic Doctor! (naturopathic.org)

Mold-literate practitioners list (drcrista.com)

AIR FILTERS

Ionizing type—Intellipure Premium Plus at pureairdoctor.com

HyperHEPA type—IQ Air at iqair.com

Incinerator type—AirFree at airfree.com

PRODUCTS (Note: Some require a doctor's prescription)

Sweetish Bitters—Gaia Herbs & Wise Woman Herbals

Glutathione Liposomal—Readisorb & Seeking Health

Resveratrol—Gaia Herbs

Liposomal Curcuma/Resveratrol—Empirical Labs

Peloid/Moor mud soak—Torf Spa at torfspa.com
Torf Czech Natural Moor Mud for Bath or Bodywrap Sachet
Torf Hévíz Natural Moor Mud for Bath or Bodywrap
(follow instructions on their website for use)

Sauna—Be cautious about FIR saunas that emit EMFs.
Offering low EMF-emmitting:
Sauna Ray (saunaray.com)
Radiant Health (radianthealthsaunas.com)

Nebulizers—NasoNeb, NasoTouch

Nasal Sprays
Fess brand Frequent Flyer
PurEssentiel brand Respiratoire
Xylitol, Xlear
NaturaNectar brand Propolis (please use this one only if others don't work—our bees are struggling so this is a precious resource)

Coffee—Bulletproof coffee
(bulletproof.com/collections/coffee)

Wine—Dry Farm Wines (dryfarmwines.com)

ACKNOWLEDGMENTS

Thank you for your enduring support:

my boys
my sweetheart from afar
my parents
my family
my friends
my teachers
my patients (who are my best teachers)
my colleagues
Leann, for…well, everything!

Kristin, for sharing your gift of translating my scrambled mind into the creation of gorgeous design work

Tabby, for convincing me to get my message out about mold

Lynda Goldman, my angel who arrived at the perfect time to guide me on the book writing and publishing process

Northern Exposure TV Series—my first exposure to environmental illness

Dr. Walter Crinnion—environmental medicine guru and inspirator

Dr. Pamela Jeanne—for infecting me with your passion for hydrotherapy

Dr. Jared Zeff—for teaching me faith in the healing power of the body

Dr. Lisa Nagy—for being the first lecturer to help me "get it" about mold

Dr. Jim Sensenig—for keeping me juiced about our medicine

The late Dr. Kim Saxe—whose mold torch I proudly carry on

Thank you for providing forums to help me on my mission to educate people on the dangers of mold.

(listed in order of appearance or publication date)

WNDA—Wisconsin Naturopathic Doctors Association (wisconsin-nd.org)

AIHM—Academy of Integrative Health & Medicine (aihm.org)

AANP—American Association of Naturopathic Physicians (naturopathic.org)

Townsend Letter (townsendletter.com)

Gaia Herbs Professional Webinar Series (gaiaprofessional.com)

ILADS—International Lyme and Associated Diseases Society (ilads.org)

Women's Health Network (womenshealthnetwork.com)

PANP—Pennsylvania Association of Naturopathic Physicians (panaturopathic.org)

Hawaii Doc Talks (events.syncopatemeetings.com/hawaii-doc-talks/)

NDNR—Naturopathic Doctor News & Review, coming soon! (ndnr.com)

Notes

Abbott, S. "Mycotoxins and Indoor Molds." Indoor Environment Connections, 2002; 3(4).

Accardi, R., H. Gruffat, C. Sirand, et al. "The mycotoxin aflatoxin B1 stimulates Epstein-Barr virus-induced B-cell transformation in in vitro and in vivo experimental models." Carcinogenesis, 2015 November; 36(11): 1440-51. doi: 10.1093/carcin/bgv142.

Akinrinmade, F. J., A. S. Akinrinde, and A. Amid. "Changes in serum cytokine levels, hepatic and intestinal morphology in aflatoxin B1-induced injury: modulatory roles of melatonin and flavonoid-rich fractions from Chromolena odorata." Mycotoxin Research, 2016 May; 32(2): 53-60. doi: 10.1007/s12550-016-0239-9.

Al-Anati, L., E. Essid, R. Reinehr, and E. Petzinger. "Silibinin protects OTA-mediated TNF-alpha release from perfused rat livers and isolated rat Kupffer cells." Molecular Nutrition & Food Research, 2009 April; 53(4): 460-6. doi: 10.1002/mnfr.200800110.

Al-Harbi, N. O., A. Nadeem, M. M. Al-Harbi, et al. "Oxidative airway inflammation leads to systemic and vascular oxidative stress in a murine model of allergic asthma." International Immunopharmacology, 2015 May; 26(1): 237-45. doi: 10.1016/j.intimp.2015.03.032.

Andersen, B., J. C. Frisvad, I. Søndergaard, et al. "Associations between fungal species and water-damaged building materials." Applied and Environmental Microbiology, 2011 June; 77(12): 4180-8. doi: 10.1128/AEM.02513-10.

Angeli, J. P., G. R. Barcelos, J. M. Serpeloni, et al. "Evaluation of the genotoxic and anti-genotoxic activities of silybin in human hepatoma cells (HepG2)." Mutagenesis, 2010 May; 25(3): 223-9. doi: 10.1093/mutage/gep064.

Araújo, A. A., M. G. de Melo, T. K. Rabelo, et al. "Review of the biological properties and toxicity of usnic acid." Natural Product Research, 2015; 29(23): 2167-80. doi: 10.1080/14786419.2015.1007455.

Batista, E. M., J. G. Doria, T. H. Ferreira-Vieira, et al. "Orchestrated activation of mGIuR5 and CB1 promotes neuroprotection." Molecular Brain, 2016 August 20; 9(1): 80. doi: 10.1186/s13041-016-0259-6.

Baxi, S. N., J. M. Portnoy, D. Larenas-Linnemann, and W. Phipatanakul. "Exposure and Health Effects of Fungi on Humans." The Journal of Allergy and Clinical Immunology: In Practice, 2016 May-June; 4(3): 396-404. doi: 10.1016/j-jaip.2016.01.008.

Behr, J., B. Degenkolb, T. Beinert, et al. "Pulmonary glutathione levels in acute episodes of Farmer's lung." American Journal of Respiratory and Critical Care Medicine, 2000 June; 161(6): 1968-71.

Behrens, M., S. Hüwel, H. J. Galla, and H. U. Humpf. "Blood-Brain Barrier Effects of the Fusarium Mycotoxins Deoxynivalenol, 3 Acetyldeoxynivalenol, and Moniliformin and Their Transfer to the Brain." PLoS One, 2015 November 23; 10(11): e0143640. doi: 10.1371/journal.pone.0143640.

Ben Salem, I., A. Prola, M. Boussabbeh, et al. "Crocin and Quercetin protect HCT116 and HEK293 cells from Zearalenone-induced apoptosis by reducing endoplasmic reticulum stress." Cell Stress and Chaperones, 2015 November; 20(6): 927-38. doi: 10.1007/s12192-015-0613-0.

Bharti, V., N. Vasudeva, and S. Kumar. "Anti-oxidant studies and anti-microbial effect of Origanum vulgare Linn in combination with standard antibiotics." Ayu, 2014 January-March; 35(1): 71-8. doi: 10.4103/0974-8520.141944.

Bloom, E., L. F. Grimsley, C. Pehrson, et al. "Molds and mycotoxins in dust from water-damaged homes in New Orleans after hurricane Katrina." Indoor Air, 2009; 19: 153-8. doi: 10.1111/j.1600-0668.2008.00574.x.

Bloom, E., E. Nyman, A. Must, et al. "Molds and mycotoxins in indoor environments—a survey in water-damaged buildings." Journal of Occupational and Environmental Hygiene, 2009 November; 6(11): 671-8. doi: 10.1080/15459620903252053.

Boeira, S. P., C. B. Filho, L. Del'Fabbro, et al. "Lycopene treatment prevents hematological, reproductive and histopathological damage induced by acute zearalenone administration in male Swiss mice." Experimental and Toxicologic Pathology, 2014 July; 66(4): 179-85. doi: 10.1016/j.etp.2014.01.002.

Borok, Z., R. Buhl, G. J. Grimes, et al. "Effect of glutathione aerosol on oxidant-antioxidant imbalance in idiopathic pulmonary fibrosis." Lancet, 1991 July 27; 338(8761): 215-6.

Brewer, J. H., D. Hooper, and S. Muralidhar. "Intranasal antifungal therapy in patients with chronic illness associated with mold and mycotoxins: an observational analysis." Global Journal of Medical Research, 2015; 15(1): 28-33.

Brewer, J. H., J. D. Thrasher, and D. Hooper. "Chronic illness associated with mold and mycotoxins: Is naso-sinus fungal biofilm a culprit?" Toxins, 2013 December 24; 6(1): 66-80. doi: 10.3390/toxins6010066.

Brewer, J.H., J. D. Thrasher, D. C. Straus, et al. "Detection of mycotoxins in patients with chronic fatigue syndrome." Toxins, 2013 April 11; 5(4): 605-17. doi: 10.3390/toxins5040605.

Brook, I. "Microbiology of chronic rhinosinusitis." European Journal of Clinical Microbiology & Infectious Diseases, 2016 July; 35(7): 1059-68. doi: 10.1007/s10096-016-2640-x.

Cantorna, M., L. Snyder, Y. Lin, and Y. Linlin. "Vitamin D and 1,25(OH)2D Regulation of T cells." Nutrients, 2015 April; 7(4): 3011-3021. doi: 10.3390/nu7043011.

Cardoso, N., C. Alviano, A. Blank, et al. "Synergism Effect of the Essential Oil from Ocimum basilicum var. Maria Bonita and Its Major Components with Fluconazole and Its Influence on Erogosterol Biosynthesis." Evidence-Based Complementary and Alternative Medicine, 2016 May 5: 5647182. doi: 10.1155/2016/5647182.

Chen, J., C. Wang, W. Lan, et al. "Gliotoxin Inhibits Proliferation and Induces Apoptosis in Colorectal Cancer Cells." Marine Drugs, 2015 October 2; 13(10):6259-73. doi: 10.3390/md13106259.

Chen, K. H., T. Gao, J. F. Pan, et al. "[Docosahexaenoic acid inhibits aflatoxin B1-induced migration and invasion in hepatocellular carcinoma cells in vitro.]" Nan Fang Yi Ke Da Xue Xue Bao, 2016 June 20; 36(7): 952-6.

Chung, Y. C., W. H. Shin, J. Y. Baek, et al. "CB2 receptor activation prevents glial-derived neurotoxic mediator production, BBB leakage and peripheral immune cell infiltration and rescues dopamine neurons in the MPTP model of Parkinson's disease." Experimental & Molecular Medicine, 2016 January 22; 48(1): e205. doi: 10.1038/emm.2015.100.

Colombo, M., A. Sangiovanni. "[Hepatocellular carcinoma]." Recenti Progressi in Medicina, 2016 July; 107(7): 386-94. doi: 10.1701/2318.24934.

Crinnion, W. Clean, Green & Lean. Hoboken, NJ: John Wiley & Sons Inc; 2010.

Curtis, L., A. Lieberman, M. Stark, et al. "Adverse Health Effects of Indoor Molds." Journal of Nutritional & Environmental Medicine, 2004 September; 14(3): 261-74. doi: 10.1080/13590840400010318.

de Carvalho, M. P., H. Weich, and W. R. Abraham. "Macrocyclic trichothecenes as antifungal and anticancer compounds." Current Medicinal Chemistry, 2016; 23(1): 23-35.

Devinsky, O., M. R. Cilio, H. Cross, et al. "Cannabidiol: pharmacology and potential therapeutic role in epilepsy and other neuropsychiatric disorders." Epilepsia, 2014 June; 55(6): 791-802. doi: 10.1111/epi.12631.

Du, K., C. Wang, P. Liu, et al. "Effects of Dietary Mycotoxins on Gut Microbiome." Protein & Peptide Letters, 2017 May 10; 24(5): 397-405. doi: 10.2174/092986652466617 0223095207.

El-Bahr, S. M. "Effect of curcumin on hepatic antioxidant enzymes activities and gene expressions in rats intoxicated with aflatoxin B1." Phytotherapy Research, 2015 January; 29(1): 134-40. doi: 10.1002/ptr.5239.

El-Bialy, B. E., E. E. Abdeen, N. B. El-Borai, and E. M. El-Diasty. "Experimental Studies on Some Immunotoxicological Aspects of Aflatoxins Containing Diet and Protective Effect of Bee Pollen Dietary Supplement." Pakistan Journal of Biological Sciences, 2016 January; 19(1): 26-35.

El-Kamary, S. S., M. D. Shardell, M. Abdel-Hamid, et al. "A randomized controlled trial to assess the safety and efficacy of silymarin on symptoms, signs and biomarkers of acute hepatitis." Phytomedicine, 2009 May; 16(5): 391-400. doi: 10.1016/j.phymed.2009.02.002.

El-Soud, N. H., M. Deabes, L. A. El-Kassem, and M. Khalil. "Chemical Composition and Antifungal Activity of Ocimum basilicum L. Essential Oil." Open Access Macedonian Journal of Medical Sciences, 2015 September 15; 3(3): 374-9. doi: 10.3889/oamjms.2015.082.

Fernández-Blanco, C., G. Font, and M. J. Ruiz. "Role of quercetin on Caco-2 cells against cytotoxic effects of alternariol and alternariol monomethyl ether." Food and Chemicak Toxicology, 2016 March; 89: 60-6. doi: 10.1016/j.fct.2016.01.011.

Fog Nielsen, K. "Mycotoxin production by indoor molds." Fungal Genetics and Biology, 2003 July; 39(2): 103-17.

Friedman, M. "Overview of antibacterial, antitoxin, antiviral, and antifungal activities of tea flavonoids and teas." Molecular Nutrition & Food Research, 2007 January; 51(1): 116-34.

Funk, R. H., and T. K. Monsees. "Effects of electromagnetic fields on cells: physiological and therapeutical approaches and molecular mechanisms of interaction. A review." Cells Tissues Organs, 2006; 182(2): 59-78. doi: 10.1159/000093061.

Gao, S. S., X. Y. Chen, R. Z. Zhu, et al. "Sulforaphane induces glutathione S-transferase isozymes which detoxify aflatoxin B(1)-8,9-epoxide in AML 12 cells." BioFactors, 2010 Jul-Aug; 36(4): 289-96. doi: 10.1002/biof.98.

Gedalia, A., T. A. Khan, A. K. Shetty, et al. "Childhood sarcoidosis: Louisiana experience." Clinical Rheumatology, 2016 July; 35(7): 1879-84. doi: 10.1007/s10067-015-2870-9.

Gholami-Ahangaran, M., N. Rangsaz, and S. Azizi. "Evaluation of turmeric (Curcuma longa) effect on biochemical and pathological parameters of liver and kidney in chicken aflatoxicosis." Pharmaceutical Biology, 2016; 54(5): 780-7. doi: 10.3109/13880209.2015.1080731.

González, R, I. Ballester, R. López-Posadas, et al. "Effects of flavonoids and other polyphenols on inflammation." Critical Reviews in Food Science and Nutrition, 2011 April; 51(4): 331-62. doi: 10.1080/10408390903584094.

Gots, R. E., N. J. Layton, and S. W. Pirages. "Indoor Health: Background Levels of Fungi." AIHA Journal, 2003; 64(4): 427-38. doi: 10.1080/15428110308984836.

Grant, R., and J. Guest. "Role of Omega-3 PUFAs in Neurobiological Health." Advances in Neurogiology, 2016; 12: 247-74. doi: 10.1007/978-3-319-28383-8_13.

Guibas, G. V., E. Spandou, S. Meditskou, et al. "N-acetylcysteine exerts therapeutic action in a rat model of allergic rhinitis." International Forum of Allergy & Rhinology, 2013 July; 3(7): 543-9. doi: 10.1002/alr.21145.

Guilford, F.T., and J. Hope. "Deficient glutathione in the pathophysiology of mycotoxin-related illness." Toxins, 2014 February 10; 6(2): 608-23. doi: 10.3390/toxins6020608.

Harms, H., B. Orlikova, S. Ji, et al. "Epipolythiodiketopiperazines from the Marine Derived Fungus Dichotomomyces cejpii with NF-kB Inhibitory Potential." Marine Drugs, 2015 August 6;13(8):4949-66. doi: 10.3390/md13084949.

Hashmi, M., A. Khan, M. Hanif, et al. "Traditional Uses, Phytochemistry, and Pharmacology of Olea europaea (Olive)." Evidence-Based Complementary and Alternative Medicine, 2015; 2015: 541581. doi: 10.1155/2015/541591.

Hawke, R. L., S. J. Schrieber, T. A. Soule, et al. "Silymarin ascending multiple oral dosing phase I study in noncirrhotic patients with chronic hepatitis C." The Journal of Clinical Pharmacology, 2010 April; 50(4): 434-49. doi: 10.1177/0091270009347475.

Herter, I., G. Geginat, H. Hof, and C. Kupfahl. "Modulation of innate and antigen-specific immune functions directed against Listeria monocytogenes by fungal toxins in vitro." Mycotoxin Research, 2014 May; 30(2): 79-87. doi: 10.1007/s12550-014-0191-5.

Hooper, D. G., V. E. Bolton, F. T. Guilford, and D. C. Straus. "Mycotoxin detection in human samples from patients exposed to environmental molds." International Journal of Molecular Sciences, 2009 April 1; 10(4): 1465-75. doi: 10.3390/ijms10041465.

Hope, J. "A review of the mechanism of injury and treatment approaches for illness resulting from exposure to water-damage buildings, mold, and mycotoxins." ScientificWorldJournal, 2013 April 18; 2013: 767482. doi: 10.1155/2013/767482.

Hope, J. H., and B. E. Hope. "A review of the diagnosis and treatment of Ochratoxin A inhalation exposure associated with human illness and kidney disease including focal segmental glomerulosclerosis." Journal of Environmental and Public Health, 2012; 2012: 835059. doi: 10.1155/2012/835059.

Hubmann, R., M. Hilgarth, S. Schnabl, et al. "Gliotoxin is a potent NOTCH2 transactivation inhibitor and efficiently induces apoptosis in chronic lymphocytic leukaemia (CLL) cells." British Journal of Haematology, 2013 March; 160(5):618-29. doi: 10.1111/bjh.12183.

Hudson, J., M. Kuo, and S. Vimalanathan. "The antimicrobial properties of cedar leaf (Thuja plicate) oil; a safe and efficient decontamination agent for buildings." International Journal of Environmental Research and Public Health, 2011 December; 8(12): 4477-87. doi: 10.3390/ijerph8124477.

Iossifova, Y. Y., J. M. Cox-Ganser, J. H. Park, et al. "Lack of respiratory improvement following remediation of a water-damaged office building." American Journal of Industrial Medicine, 2011 April; 54(4): 269-77. doi: 10.1002/ajim.20910.

Iram, W., T. Anjum, M. Iqbal, et al. "Structural analysis and biological toxicity of Aflatoxins B1 and B2 degradation products following detoxification by Ocimum basilicum and Cassia fistula aqueous extracts." Frontiers in Microbiology, 2016 July 14; 7: 1105. doi: 10.3389/fmicb.2016.01105.

Jarolim, K., G. Del Favero, G. Pahlke, et al. "Activation of the Nrf2-ARE pathway by the Alternaria alternata mycotoxins altertoxin I and II." Archives of Toxicology, 2016 May 13. doi:10.1007/s00204-016-1726-7.

Jia, Q., H. R. Zhou, M. Bennink, and J. J. Pestka. "Docosahexaenoic acid attenuates mycotoxin-induced immunoglobulin a nephropathy, interleukin-6 transcription, and mitogen-activated protein kinase phosphorylation in mice." The Journal of Nutrition, 2004 December; 134(12): 3343-9.

Jones, G. L., C. G. Lane, E. E. Daniel, and P. M. O'Byrne. "Release of epithelium-derived relaxing factor after ozone inhalation in dogs." Journal of Applied Physiology, 1988 September; 65(3): 1238-43.

Karaman, M., H. Ozen, M. Tuzcu, et al. "Pathological, biochemical and haematological investigations on the protective effect of alpha-lipoic acid in experimental aflatoxin toxicosis in chicks." British Poultry Science, 2010 February; 51(1): 132-41. doi: 10.1080/00071660903401839.

Kaya, I., N. Yigit, and M. Benli. "Antimicrobial Activity of Various Extracts of Ocimum Basilicum L. and Observation of the Inhibition Effect on Bacterial Cells by Use of Scanning Electron Microscopy." African Journal of Traditional, Complementary and Alternative Medicines, 2008 June 18; 5(4): 363-369.

Khatoon, A., M. Zargham Khan, A. Khan, et atl. "Amelioration of Ochratoxin A-incuded immunotoxic effects by silymarin and Vitamin E in White Leghorn cockerels." Journal of Immunotoxicology, 2013 January-March; 10(1): 25-31. doi: 10.3109/1547691X.2012.686533.

Knudsen, P. B., B. Hanna, S. Ohl, et al. "Chaetoglobosin A preferentially induces apoptosis in chronic lymphocytic leukemia cells by targeting the cytoskeleton." Leukemia, 2014 June; 28(6): 1289-98. doi: 10.1038/leu.2013.360.

Kostek, H., J. Szponar, M. Tchórz, et al. "[Silibinin and its hepatoprotective action from the perspective of a toxicologist.]" Przegl Lek, 2012; 69(8): 541-3.

Kőszegi, T., and M. Poór. "Ochratoxin A: Molecular Interactions, Mechanisms of Toxicity and Prevention at the Molecular Level." Toxins, 2016 April 15; 8(4): 111. doi: 10.3390/toxins8040111.

Kumari, I., M. Ahmed, and Y. Akhter. "Multifaceted impact of trichothecene metabolites on plant-microbe interactions and human health." Applied Microbiology and Biotechnology, 2016 July; 100(13): 5759-71. doi: 10.1007/s00253-016-7599-0.

Kupfahl, C., G. Geginat, and H. Hof. "Gliotoxin-mediated suppression of innate and adaptive immune functions directed against Listeria monocytogenes." Medical Mycology, 2006 November; 44(7): 591-9.

Kupski, L., M. Freitas, D. Ribeiro, et al. "Ochratoxin A activates neutrophils and kills these cells through necrosis, an effect eliminated through its conversion into ochratoxin α." Toxicology, 2016 August 10; 368-369: 91-102. doi: 10.1016/j.tox.2016.09.001.

Lai, F. N., J. Y. Ma, J. C. Liu, et al. "The influence of N-acetyl-l-cysteine on damage of porcine oocyte exposed to zearalenone in vitro." Toxicology and Applied Pharmacology, 2015 December 1; 289(2): 341-8. doi: 10.1016/j.taap.2015.09.010.

Li, B., Y. Gao, G.O. Rankin, et al. "Chaetoglobosin K induces apoptosis and G2 cell cycle arrest through p53-dependent pathway in cisplatin-resistant ovarian cancer cells." Cancer Letters, 2015 January 28; 356(2 Pt B): 418-33. doi: 10.1016/j.canlet.2014.09.023.

Li, Y., Q. G. Ma, L. H. Zhao, et al. "Effects of lipoic acid on immune function, the antioxidant defense system, and inflammation-related genes expression of broiler chickens fed aflatoxin contaminated diets." International Journal of Molecular Sciences, 2014 April 2; 15(4): 5649-62. doi: 10.3390/ijms15045649.

Liang, N., F. Wang., X. Peng., et al. "Effect of Sodium Selenite on Pathological Changes and Renal Functions in Broilers Fed a Diet Containing Aflatoxin B_1." International Journal of Environmental Research and Public Health, 2015 September 9; 12(9): 11196-208. doi: 10.3390/ijerph120911196.

Liu, L. T., G. J. Zheng, W. G. Zhang, et al. "[Clinical study on treatment of carotid atherosclerosis with extraction of polygon cuspidate rhizome et radix and crataegi fructus: a randomized controlled trial.]" Zhonggou Zhong Yao Za Zhi, 2014 March; 39(6): 1115-9.

Lou, H., B. Li, Z. Li, et al. "Chaetoglobosin K inhibits tumor angiogenesis through down regulation of vascular epithelial growth factor-binding hypoxia-inducible factor 1a." Anticancer Drugs, 2013 August; 24(7): 715-24. doi: 10.1097/CAD.0b013e3283627a0b.

Ma, Q., Y. Li, Y. Fan, et al. "Molecular Mechanisms of Lipoic Acid Protection against Aflatoxin B_1-Induced Liver Oxidative Damage and Inflammatory Responses in Broilers." Toxins, 2015 December 14; 7(12): 5435-47. doi: 10.3390/toxins7124879.

Malir, F., V. Ostry, A. Pfohl-Leszkowicz, et al. "Ochratoxin A: 50 Years of Research." Toxins, 2016 July 4; 8(7). pii: E191. doi: 10.3390/toxins8070191.

Marchese, A., I. E. Orhan, M. Daglia, et al. "Antibacterial and antifungal activities of thymol: A brief review of the literature." Food Chemistry, 2016 November 1; 210: 402-14. doi: 10.1016/j.foodchem.2016.04.111.

Maresca, M., R. Mahfoud, N. Garmy, and J. Fantini. "The mycotoxin deoxynivalenol affects nutrient absorption in human intestinal epithelial cells." The Journal of Nutrition, 2002 September; 132(9): 2723-31.

Mary, V. S., A. Valdehita, J. M Navas, et al. "Effects of aflatoxin B_1, fumonisin B_1 and their mixture on the aryl hydrocarbon receptor and cytochrome P450 1A induction." Food and Chemical Toxicology, 2015 January; 75: 104-11. doi: 10.1016/j.fct.2014.10.030.

Masoko, P., and D. M. Makgapeetja. "Antibacterial, antifungal and antioxidant activity of Olea africana against pathogenic yeast and nosocomial pathogens." BMC Complementary Alternative Medicine, 2015 November 17; 15: 409. doi: 10.1186/s12906-015-0941-8.

Matters, G. L., J. F. Harms, C. McGovern, et al. "The opioid antagonist naltrexone improves murine inflammatory bowel disease." Journal of Immunotoxicology, 2008 April; 5(2): 179-87. doi: 10.1080/15476910802131469.

Mayurasakorn, K., Z. V. Niatsetskaya, S. A. Sosunov, et al. "DHA but Not EPA Emulsions Preserve Neurological and Mitochondrial Function after Brain Hypoxia-Ischemia in Neonatal Mice." PLoS One, 2016 August 11; 11(8): e0160870. doi: 10.1371/journal.pone.0160870.

Meki, A. R., S. K. Abdel-Ghaffar, and I. El-Gibaly. "Aflatoxin B1 induces apoptosis in rat liver: protective effect of melatonin." Neuro Endocrinology Letters, 2001 December; 22(6): 417-26.

Meki, A. R., and A. A. Hussein. "Melatonin reduces oxidative stress induced by ochratoxin A in rat liver and kidney." Comparative Biochemistry and Physiology Part C: Toxicology & Pharmacology, 2001 November; 130(3): 305-13.

Mikaili, P., S. Maadirad, M. Moloudizargari, et al. "Therapeutic Uses and Pharmacological Properties of Garlic, Shallot, and Their Biologically Active Compounds." Iranian Journal of Basic Medical Sciences, 2013 October; 16(10): 1031-1048.

Mitropoulou, G., E. Fitsiou, E. Stavropoulou, et al. "Composition, antimicrobial, antioxidant, and anti proliferative activity of Origanum dictamnus (dittany) essential oil." Microbial Ecology in Health and Disease, 2015; 26: 10.3402/mehd.v26.26543.

Published online 2015 May 6. doi: 10.3402/mehd.v26.26543.

Mohammadpour, H., E. Moghimipour, I. Rasooli, et al. "Chemical Composition and Antifungal Activity of Cuminum cyminum L. Essential Oil From Alborz Mountain Against Aspergillus species." Jundishapur Journal of Natural Pharmaceutical Products, 2012 Spring; 7(2): 50-5.

Morimitsu, Y., Y. Nakagawa, K. Hayashi, et al. "A sulforaphane analogue that potently activates the Nrf2-dependent detoxification pathway." Journal of Biological Chemistry, 2002 February 1; 277(5): 3456-63. doi: 10.1074/jbc.M110244200.

Muminov, A. I., and N. Zh. Khushvakova. "[Ozone therapy in patients with chronic purulent frontal sinusitis]." Vestn Otorinolaringol, 2002; (6): 46.

Nagata, K., K. I. Hirai, J. Koyama, et al. "Antimicrobial Activity of Novel Furanonaphthoquinone Analogs." Antimicrobial Agents and Chemotherapy, 1998 March; 42(3): 700-2.

Ninković, J., and S. Roy. "Role of the mu opioid receptor in opioid modulation of immune function." Amino Acids, 2013 July; 45(1): 9-24. doi: 10.1007/s00726-011-1163-0.

Nithyanand, P., R. M. Beema Shafreen, S. Muthamil, and S. Karutha Pandian. "Usnic acid, a lichen secondary metabolite inhibits Group A Streptococcus biofilms." Antonie Van Leeuwenhoek, 2015 January; 107(1): 263-72. doi: 10.1007/s10482-014-0324-z.

Nithyanand, P., R. M. Beema Shafreen, S. Muthamil, and S. Karutha Pandian. "Usnic acid inhibits biofilm formation and virulent morphological traits of Candida albicans." Microbiological Research, 2015 October; 179: 20-8. doi: 10.1016/j.micres.2015.06.009.

Ohtsubo, K., M. Saito, S. Sekita, et al. "Acute toxic effects of chaetoglobosin A, a new cytochalasan compound produced by Chaetomium globosum, on mice and rats." Japanese Journal of Experimental Medicine, 1978 April; 48(2): 105-10.

Pahlke, G., C. Tiessen, K. Domnanich, et al. "Impact of Alternaria toxins on CYP1A1 expression in different human tumor cells and relevance for genotoxicity." Toxicology Letters, 2016 January 5; 240(1): 93-104. doi: 10.1016/j.toxlet.2015.10.003.

Paraschiv, B., A. C. Sellier, C. Diaconu, and R. Bernard. "Sarcoidosis and Aspergillosis: case presentation." Pneumologia, 2015 Jul-Sep; 64(3): 50-4.

Patel, K. R., C. Andreadi, R. G. Britton, et al. "Sulfate metabolites provide an intracellular pool for resveratrol generation and induce autophagy with senescence." Science Translational Medicine, 2013 October 2; 5(205): 205ra133. doi: 10.1126/scitranslmed.3005870.

Patwardhan, J., and P. Bhatt. "Flavonoids Derived from Abelmoschus esculentus Attenuates UV-B Induced Cell Damage in Human Dermal Fibroblasts Through Nrf2-ARE Pathway." Pharmacognosy Magazine, 2016 May; 12(Suppl 2): S129-38. doi: 10.4103/0973-1296.182175.

Pereira, E. M., T. de B. Machado, I. C. R. Leal, et al. "Tabebuia avellanedae naphthoquinones: activity against methicillin-resistant staphylococcal strains, cytotoxic activity and in vivo dermal irritability analysis." Annals of Clinical Microbiology and Antimicrobials, 2006; 5: 5. doi: 10.1186/1476-0711-5-5.

Periasamy, R., I. G. Kalal, R. Krishnaswamy, and V. Viswanadha. "Quercetin protects human peripheral blood mononuclear cells from OTA-induced oxidative stress, genotoxicity, and inflammation." Environmental Toxicology, 2016 July; 31(7): 855-65. doi: 10.1002/tox.22096.

Petrov, G. M., B. P. Kudriavtsev, and I. I. Akulich. "[The efficacy of using ozone preparations in the combined treatment of paranasal sinusitis]." Voen Med Zh, 1996 December; 317(12): 26-8, 80.

Pitkäranta, M., T. Meklin, A. Hyvärinen, et al. "Molecular profiling of fungal communities in moisture damaged buildings before and after remediation—a comparison of culture-dependent and culture-independent methods." BMC Microbiology, 2011 October 21; 11: 235.

Pizzorno, J. "Is Mold Toxicity Really a Problem for Our Patients? Part I-Respiratory Conditions." Integrative Medicine: A Clinician's Journal (Encinitas), 2016 April; 15(2): 6-10.

Poursky, J. "The treatment of pulmonary diseases and respiratory-related conditions with inhaled (nebulized or aerosolized) glutathione." Evidence-based Complementary and Alternative Medicine, 2008 March; 5(1): 27-35. doi: 10.1093/ecam/nem040.

Raghubeer, S., S. Nagiah, A. Phulukdaree, and A. Chuturgoon. "The phytoalexin resveratrol ameliorates Ochratoxin A toxicity in human embryonic kidney (HEK293) cells." Journal of Cellular Biochemistry, 2015 December; 116(12): 2947-55. doi: 10.1002/jcb.25242.

Ramyaa, P., R. Krishnaswamy, and V. V. Padma. "Quercetin modulates OTA-induced oxidative stress and redox signalling in HepG2 cells - up regulation of Nrf2 expression and down regulation of NF-κB and COX-2." Biochimica et Biophysica Acta, 2014 January; 1840(1): 681-92. doi: 10.1016/j.bbagen.2013.10.024.

Rasooli, I., M. H. Fakoor, D. Yadegarinia, et al. "Antimycotoxigenic characteristics of Rosmarinus officinalis and Trachyspermum copticum L. essential oils." International Journal of Food Microbiology, 2008 February 29; 122(1-2): 135-9. doi: 10.1016/j.ijfoodmicro.2007.11.048.

Reasor, M. J., G. K. Adams III, J. K. Brooks, and R. J. Rubin. "Enrichment of albumin in IgG in the airway secretions of dogs breathing ozone." Journal of Environmental Science and Health, Part C, 1979; 13(4): 335-46.

Reeves, E.P., T. Murphy, P. Daly, and K. Kavanagh. "Amphotericin B enhances the synthesis and release of the immunosuppressive agent gliotoxin from the pulmonary pathogen Aspergillus fumigatus." Journal of Medical Microbiology, 2004 August; 53(Pt 8): 719-25. doi: 10.1099/jmm.0.45626-0.

Rip, J., L. Chen, R. Hartman, et al. "Glutathione PEGylated liposomes: pharmacokinetics and delivery of cargo across the blood-brain barrier in rats." Journal of Drug Targeting, 2014 June; 22(5): 460-7. doi: 10.3109/1061186X.2014.888070.

Rogawansamy, S., S. Gaskin, M. Taylor, and D. Pisaniello. "An Evaluation of Antifungal Agents for the Treatment of Fungal Contamination in Indoor Air Environments." International Journal of Environmental Research and Public Health, 2015 June; 12(6): 6319-6332. doi: 10.3390/ijerph120606319.

Saad-Hussein, A., E. M. Shahy, W. Shaheen, et al. "Comparative Hepatotoxicity of Aflatoxin B1 among Workers Exposed to Different Organic Dust with Emphasis on Polymorphism Role of Glutathione S-Transferase Gene." Open Access Macedonian Journal of Medical Sciences, 2016 June 15; 4(2): 312-8. doi: 10.3889/oamjms.2016.051.

Schäfer, G., and C. Kaschula. "The Immunomodulation and Anti-Inflammatory Effects of Garlic Organosulfur Compounds in Cancer Chemoprevention." Anti-Cancer Agents Medicinal Chemistry, 2014 February; 14(2): 233-240. doi: 10.2174/18715206113136660370.

Scharf, D.M., P. Chankhamjon, K. Scherlach, et al. "Epidithiodiketopiperazine biosynthesis: a four-enzyme cascade converts glutathione conjugates into transannular disulfide bridges." Angewandte Chemie International Edition English, 2013 October 11; 52(42): 11092-5. doi: 10.1002/anie.201305059.

Segvić Klarić, M., I. Kosalec, J. Mastelić, et al. "Antifungal activity of thyme (Thymus vulgaris L.) essential oil and thymol against moulds from damp dwellings." Letters in Applied Microbiology, 2007 January; 44(1): 36-42.

Sen, B., and A. Asan. "Fungal flora in indoor and outdoor air of different residential houses in Tekirdag City (Turkey): seasonal distribution and relationship with climatic factors." Environmental Monitoring and Assessment, 2009 April; 151(1-4): 209-19. doi: 10.1007/s10661-008-0262-1.

Sharifzadeh, A., and H. Shokri. "Antifungal activity of essential oils from Iranian plants against fluconazole-resistant and fluconazole-susceptible Candida albicans." Avicenna Journal of Phytomedicine, 2016 March-April; 6(2): 215-22.

Shi, D., S. Liao, S. Guo, et al. "Protective effects of selenium on aflatoxin B1-induced mitochondrial permeability transition, DNA damage, and histological alterations in duckling liver." Biological Trace Element Research, 2015 February; 163(1-2): 162-8. doi: 10.1007/s12011-014-0189-z.

Shimono, J., Y. Tsutsumi, and H. Ohigashi. "[Acute renal tubular damage caused by disseminated Trichosporon infection in primary myelofibrosis]. Rinsho Ketsueko, 2015 January; 56(1): 21-4. doi: 10.11406/rinketsu.56.21.

Singhal, D., A. J. Psaltis, A. Foreman, and P. J. Wormald. "The impact of biofilms on outcomes after endoscopic sinus surgery." American Journal of Rhinology and Allergy, 2010 May-June; 24(3): 169-74. doi: 10.2500/ajra.2010.24.3462.

Smith, J., D. Field, S. Bingaman, et al. "Safety and Tolerability of Low Dose Naltrexone Therapy in Children with Moderate to Severe Crohn's Disease: A Pilot Study." Journal of Clinical Gastoenterology, 2013 April; 47(4): 339-345. doi: 10.1097/MCG.0b013e3182702f2b.

Soltan-Sharifi, M. S., M. Mojtahedzadeh, A. Najafi, et al. "Improvement by N-acetylcysteine of acute respiratory distress syndrome through increasing intracellular glutathione, and extracellular thiol molecules and anti-oxidant power: evidence for underlying toxicological mechanisms." Human & Experimental Toxicology, 2007 September; 26(9): 697-703.

Souza, M. A., S. Johann, L. A. R. Lima, et al. "The antimicrobial activity of lapachol and its thiosemicarbazone and semicarbazone derivatives." Memórias do Instituto Oswaldo Cruz, 2013 May; 108(3): 342-351. doi: 10.1590/S0074-02762013000300013.

Stanley, W. C., R. J. Khairallah, and E. R. Dabkowski. "Update on lipids and mitochondrial function: impact of dietary n-3 polyunsaturated fatty acids." Current Opinion in Clinical Nutrition and Metabolic Care, 2012 March; 15(2): 122-6. doi: 10.1097/MCO.0b013e32834fdaf7.

Su, Z. Q., Z. Z. Mo, J. B. Liao, et al. "Usnic acid protects LPS-induced acute lung injury in mice through attenuating inflammatory responses and oxidative stress." International Immunopharmacology, 2014 October; 22(2): 371-8. doi: 10.1016/j.intimp.2014.06.043.

Sun, Y., K. Takada, Y. Takemoto, et al. "Gliotoxin analogues from a marine-derived fungus, Penicillium sp., and their cytotoxic and histone methyltransferase inhibitory activities." Journal of Natural Products, 2012 January 27; 75(1):111-4. doi: 10.1021/np200740e.

Sung, S. A., G.J. Ko, J. Y. Kim, et al. "Desquamative interstitial pneumonia associated with concurrent cytomegalovirus and Aspergillus pneumonia in renal transplant recipient." Nephrology Dialysis Transplantation, 2005 March; 20(3): 635-8.

Sutken, E., E. Aral, F. Ozdemir, et al. "Protective role of melatonin and coenzyme Q10 in ochratoxin A toxicity in rat liver and kidney." International Journal of Toxicology, 2007 Jan-Feb; 26(1): 81-7.

Täubel, M., M. Sulyok, V. Vishwanath, et al. "Co-occurence of toxic bacterial and fungal secondary metabolites in moisture-damaged indoor environments." Indoor Air, 2011 October; 21(5): 368-75. doi: 10.1111/j.1600-0668.2011.00721.x.

Thrasher, J.D., and S. Crawley. "The biocontaminants and complexity of damp indoor spaces: more than what meets the eyes." Toxicology and Industrial Health, 2009 Oct-Nov; 25(9-10): 583-615. doi: 10.1177/0748233709348386.

Tuli, H. S., S. S. Sandhu, and A. K. Sharma. "Pharmacological and therapeutic potential of Cordyceps with special reference to Cordycepin." Biotech, 2014 February; 4(1): 1-12. doi: 10.1007/s13205-013-0121-9.

Tuuminen, T., and K. S. Rinne. "Severe Sequelae to Mold-Related Illness as Demonstrated in Two Finnish Cohorts." Frontiers in Immunology, 2017 April 3; 8: 382. doi: 10.3389/fimmu.2017.00382.

Vojdani, A., A. W. Campbell, A. Kashanian, and E. Vojdani. "Antibodies against molds and mycotoxins following exposure to toxigenic fungi in water-damaged building." Archives of Environmental Health, 2003 June; 58(6): 324-36.

Wagner, J. G., S. J. Van Dyken, J. R. Wierenga, et al. "Ozone exposure enhances endotoxin-induced mucous cell metaplasia in rat pulmonary airways. Toxicological Sciences, 2003 August; 74(2): 437-46.

Wang, L., P. Qiu, X. F. Long, et al. "Comparative analysis of chemical constituents, antimicrobial and antioxidant activities of ethylacetate extracts of Polygonum cuspidatum and its endophytic actinomycete, Streptomyces sp. A0916." Chinese Journal of Natural Medicines, 2016 February; 14(2): 117-123. doi: 10.1016/S1875-5364(16)60004-3.

Wei, R., and S. Christakos. "Mechanisms Underlying the Regulation of Innate and Adaptive Immunity by Vitamin D." Nutrients, 2015 October; 7(10): 8251-8260. doi: 10.3390/nu7105392.

Yang, Q., L. Shi, K. Huang, and W. Xu. "Protective effect of N-acetylcysteine against DNA damage and S-phase arrest induced by ochratoxin A in human embryonic kidney cells (HEK-293)." Food and Chemical Toxicology, 2014 August; 70: 40-7. doi: 10.1016/j.fct.2014.04.039.

Yin, S., Y. Zhang, R. Gao, et al. "The immunomodulatory effects induced by dietary Zearalenone in pregnant rats." Immunopharmacology and Immunotoxicology, 2014 June; 36(3): 187-94. doi: 10.3109/08923973.2014.909847.

Yoshinari, T., A. Yaguchi, N. Takahashi-Ando, et al. "Spiroethers of German chamomile inhibit production of aflatoxin G and trichothecene mycotoxin by inhibiting cytochrome P450 monooxygenases involved in their biosynthesis." FEMS Microbiology Letters, 2008 July; 284(2): 184-90. doi: 10.1111/j.1574-6968.2008.01195.x.

Zhang, N. Y., M. Qi, L. Zhao, et al. "Curcumin Prevents Aflatoxin B_1 Hepatoxicity by Inhibition of Cytochrome P450 Isozymes in Chick Liver." Toxins, 2016 November 10; 8(11).

Zhang, X., B. Sahlberg, G. Wieslander, et al. "Dampness and moulds in workplace buildings: associations with incidence and remission of sick building syndrome (SBS) and biomarkers of inflammation in a 10 year follow-up study." Science of Total Environment, 2012 July 15; 430: 75-81.

Index